THE

PREPPER'S

POCKET COMPANION

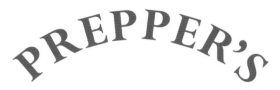

THE
PREPPER'S
POCKET COMPANION

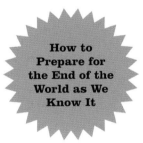

How to
Prepare for
the End of the
World as We
Know It

Kate Rowinski

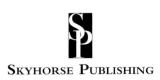

SKYHORSE PUBLISHING

Skyhorse Publishing books may be purchased in bulk at special discounts for sales promotion, corporate gifts, fund-raising, or educational purposes. Special editions can also be created to specifications. For details, contact the Special Sales Department, Skyhorse Publishing, 307 West 36th Street, 11th Floor, New York, NY 10018 or info@skyhorsepublishing.com.

Skyhorse® and Skyhorse Publishing® are registered trademarks of Skyhorse Publishing, Inc.®, a Delaware corporation.

www.skyhorsepublishing.com

10 9 8 7 6 5 4 3 2

Library of Congress Cataloging-in-Publication Data is available on file.

ISBN: 978-1-62087-261-1

Printed in China

Contents

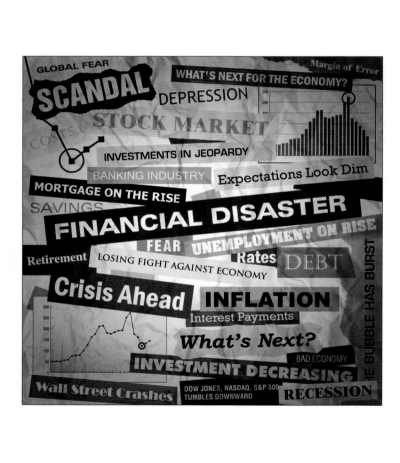

Introduction

IN THIS UNCERTAIN DAY AND AGE, IT SEEMS THAT potential disasters are around every corner. Wild weather, the threat of terrorism and pandemics, economic concerns; it is easy to feel that you and your family could fall victim at any moment. What if you lose power or the water is shut off? What if you lose your income? Could you feed your family for a day, a week, even a month? What if access to grocery stores was unavailable? Do you have a way to store and cook food in your own home?

In this world of fast food and easy access to almost anything, it may be hard to imagine a world of scarcity. But the reality is, scarcity can happen in an instant. A large tree falling on a road may keep you from the store for a day. A power outage may keep the stores closed for a week. Job loss may prevent you from shopping for three months or more.

Janice and David have a lovely home on a wooded lot. They have big screen TVs and a wonderful backyard full of great furniture, along with Mike's boat and the family's jet skis. They have full-time jobs, rely heavily on take-out food, and pick up their kids on the way home from work. Their kitchen has a sleek and modern electric stove, but Janice "doesn't cook." In fact, if you look in the cupboards, you may not find much more than a lonely pudding box and some leftover pasta noodles. They may look like they are living the American dream, but they have no idea just how close to the edge they really are. They are mortgaged to the hilt and have two car payments and four credit cards going all the time. Janice has great shoes and a nice wardrobe, but she would be hard-pressed to weather a three-day ice storm at home with her family of four. And if one of them lost a job, their savings wouldn't cover expenses for a month.

Next door, Lisa and Mike have a nice home too. But there is a big garden in the backyard, and an installed generator neatly tucked behind the garage. In the basement is a pantry stocked with several months' worth of food, batteries, and water. Mike's garage is well-organized, and he keeps his tools, chainsaw, and vehicles in top condition. The kitchen has a good gas stove, and Mike has installed a wood insert into the fireplace. He keeps a nice supply of firewood out near the shed. Low-flow toilets are installed in every bathroom. Mike and Lisa keep a weather radio on their bedside table and have a small fireproof safe for important papers, valuables, and cash. Inside each closet is a small pack labeled with the name of each member of the family. The kids know where these are and also keep laminated cards with family names and numbers in their school backpacks. If you could see inside their bank accounts, you would see a streamlined system. The mortgage isn't paid off, yet. But there are no credit card bills, their used cars are paid off, and Lisa's paycheck goes straight to savings.

So . . . which one of these families is "crazy"?

The reality is that you don't have to be a doomsday believer or a radical survivalist to be a prepper. In fact, the idea of *not* having an emergency plan and a backup supply of food and water should be as nonsensical to you as not having a tank of gas or extra batteries.

Rather than allowing the specter of disaster to loom in the back of your mind, there are simple steps you can take to make sure that your family's basic needs can be taken care of in case of an emergency.

Planning ahead provides the following benefits:

A Powerful Insurance Policy

Pre-planning is the most powerful of all bank accounts, allowing you to get through any lean times without desperation or handouts. Knowing that you have what you need no matter what happens can give you peace of mind that no homeowner's policy could ever provide.

A Sense of Self-Sufficiency

Knowing that you can take care of yourself and your family has a powerful effect on your psychological state. Taken even further, understanding how to live off the grid, take care of yourself without the conventions of civilization, and grow and preserve your own food will give your family greater appreciation for where their food comes from and a sense of gratitude for what they have.

Helping Others

Did you know the average family has less than a week's worth of food in their kitchen right now? And worse yet, if there was no power, many people wouldn't even know how to cook it! Your emergency plan will not only help keep your family safe, it may allow you to help others.

There are several useful websites and books on the topic of prepping and what to do in any emergency. *The Prepper's Pocket Companion* will give you tips, ideas, and guidance that will prepare you for almost any disaster, and knowing what to do ahead of time is always a great idea so you are not left helpless and vulnerable. It's also worth checking out Arthur Bradley's *Handbook to Practical Disaster Preparedness for the Family* and *The Disaster Preparedness Handbook*, as well as Zion Prepper's *The Prepper Handbook* for more tips and information on this topic.

Not long ago, a hurricane knocked out power to our area, taking down trees that prevented us from getting out for a few days. We were astonished to learn that most of our neighbors were not prepared to do something as simple as heating a can of beans. They could have gotten by on cereal or cheese and crackers for a couple of days. But many relied entirely on electric ranges or had outdoor grills that were out of propane. Worst of all, many had no emergency water stored. It's not that they were completely *without* resources; they just didn't have a plan.

What could have been a very uncomfortable situation turned into a party. Our chainsaw was ready to go, so the guys spent a couple of days clearing trees and opening up the road. People contributed food out of their now-useless freezers, and our emergency cooking plan fed the whole neighborhood for three days. We distributed gallons of drinking water, and a neighbor with a swimming pool supplied water for toilets. At night, we sat together around an outdoor fire, drinking beer and laughing at ourselves for not doing it more often!

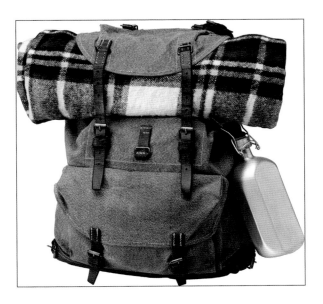

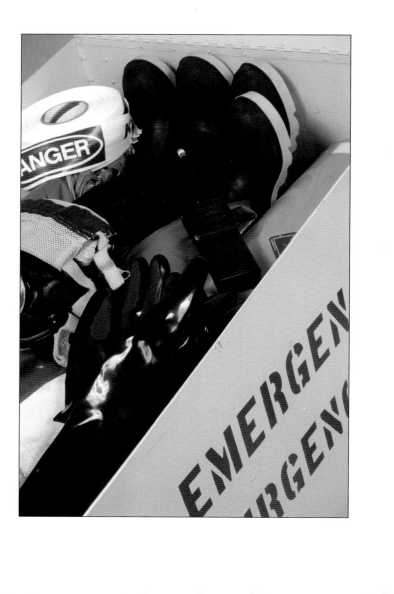

Step 1

Make a Plan!

WILL YOU BE READY IF AN EMERGENCY STRIKES? Have you thought about where to meet with your family, how you'll communicate, what resources you have for heating and transportation, and how to handle the basic functions of your home?

If not, take the time now to create your plan and walk the entire family through it. It's not enough for you to know what to do; other members of the household need to know too!

Many of us who were around on 9/11 realized after the fact just how vulnerable we were when it came to reaching out to family and friends in the middle of an emergency. Phone lines may be jammed, networks may be down, and confusion can quickly turn into panic.

With work, school, and a myriad of other activities, chances are that your family may not be together if a disaster strikes. That's why it is so important to plan in advance. Get your family together and discuss your emergency plan.

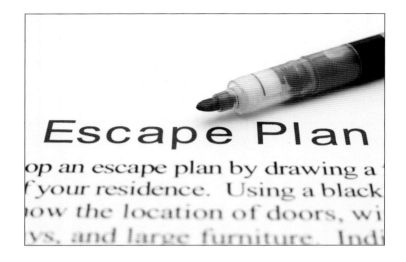

op an escape plan by drawing a
f your residence. Using a black
ow the location of doors, wi
ws, and large furniture. Indi

How will you know if there is an emergency?

State and local agencies may have alerts available that you can register for simply by providing your email address. Likewise, the National Oceanic and Atmospheric Administration (NOAA, www.noaa.gov) issues regular weather alerts.

What is your safe place?

If your home is not an option due to storms or fire, agree on somewhere else to meet that everyone in the family is familiar

Get a Weather Radio

If you are in an area where weather emergencies can strike suddenly, a weather radio will alert you to dangerous weather approaching. Weather radios broadcast NOAA's National Weather Service forecasts, watches, and warnings over a network of more than 1,000 stations.

The presence of a weather radio is especially comforting after dark, and many people keep the radio near their bed for nighttime alerts. Weather radios make a loud noise when there is a threat of bad weather anywhere in the listening area. Most are programmable so that you can tune it to only alert when the threat is in your immediate location. Most can be plugged in to a regular household outlet and have a provision for battery power as well, so make sure to keep the appropriate size batteries in your storage.

If a WATCH is announced, it means that conditions are right for the development of bad weather. Be alert and monitor conditions. Make sure you are ready for power outages, and make sure animals are inside.

If a WARNING is announced, it means that bad weather has been seen on the radar, and is occurring or imminent in your area. Take shelter immediately.

with. Include the neighbors in your plan. Have safe houses identified for your children to go to in case parents are unable to get home.

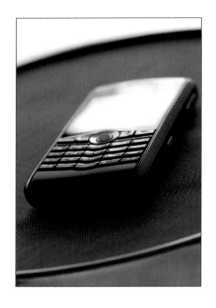

How will you communicate?

Be sure every member of your family carries important phone numbers and has a cell phone, coins, or a prepaid phone card to call their emergency contacts.

Having mobile phone service is not enough. In an emergency, phone lines are often jammed, so phone service may not be available. Text messages can often get through when a phone call cannot. Chances are that you may get information through the modern day version of the jungle drum beat—your text messages. Messages can spread like wildfire when emergencies strike. Right after an earthquake hit the East Coast, in spite of jammed phone lines, I knew in the span of only a few minutes the status of my home in the country, how the horses reacted, where my son was, and whether my friend had felt it in Boston. I was able to get a friend to check on my dogs and connect someone whose house was damaged with emergency housing.

Set up an emergency chain for your family and friends to communicate with each other. If one tells two, and two tells four, soon you will have made connections and initiated plans. Make sure everyone in the family knows how to use text messaging.

In a local emergency, it is often easier to call out of state than it is to call across town. Identify a friend or relative who lives out of state that everyone can notify that they are safe.

If you have a cell phone, program your emergency contact as "ICE" (In Case of Emergency) in your phone. If you are in an accident, emergency personnel will check for an ICE listing in your contacts in order to get ahold of someone you know. Make sure to tell your family and friends that you've listed them as emergency contacts.

Teach children to call 911.

Keep a collar, license, and ID on your dog at all times.

Write down your plan and keep a copy of it in your safe or fireproof box, so you can access it in the event of a disaster. Adults should keep a copy in their wallets or handbags, and children can have a copy in a school pack or taped to the inside of a notebook.

How much cash do you need?

Ask any expert about cash reserves and their answer will be about the same. Keep enough for three to six months of expenses readily available. Put this money in a regular savings account, not locked up in a CD or other non liquid account where

Ready
Prepare. Plan. Stay Informed. ®

Family Emergency Plan

Make sure your family has a plan in case of an emergency. Before an emergency happens, sit down together and decide how you will get in contact with each other, where you will go and what you will do in an emergency. Keep a copy of this plan in your emergency supply kit or another safe place where you can access it in the event of a disaster.

Out-of-Town Contact Name: Telephone Number:

Email:

Neighborhood Meeting Place: Telephone Number:

Regional Meeting Place: Telephone Number:

Evacuation Location: Telephone Number:

Fill out the following information for each family member and keep it up to date.

Name: Social Security Number:
Date of Birth: Important Medical Information:

Name: Social Security Number:
Date of Birth: Important Medical Information:

Name: Social Security Number:
Date of Birth: Important Medical Information:

Name: Social Security Number:
Date of Birth: Important Medical Information:

Name: Social Security Number:
Date of Birth: Important Medical Information:

Name: Social Security Number:
Date of Birth: Important Medical Information:

Write down where your family spends the most time: work, school and other places you frequent. Schools, daycare providers, workplaces and apartment buildings should all have site-specific emergency plans that you and your family need to know about.

Work Location One   School Location One
Address: Address:
Phone Number: Phone Number:
Evacuation Location: Evacuation Location:

Work Location Two   School Location Two
Address: Address:
Phone Number: Phone Number:
Evacuation Location: Evacuation Location:

Work Location Three   School Location Three
Address: Address:
Phone Number: Phone Number:
Evacuation Location: Evacuation Location:

Other place you frequent   Other place you frequent
Address: Address:
Phone Number: Phone Number:
Evacuation Location: Evacuation Location:

Important Information	Name	Telephone Number	Policy Number
Doctor(s):			
Other:			
Pharmacist:			
Medical Insurance:			
Homeowners/Rental Insurance:			
Veterinarian/Kennel (for pets):			

withdrawing early will cost you a penalty. Calculate your total bills and other essential expenses such as food and gas, and use that as your baseline. You can round up or down, based on your own comfort level. But remember, liquid assets don't earn much interest, so don't go overboard and keep all your assets liquid.

As to actual cash, we use the three-day rule. We try to keep enough cash in our home safe to get by for three days in case we have to leave the house suddenly due to a fire or other natural disaster. The amount of money should be enough to cover food, gas, hotel rooms, or other emergency needs such as extra clothes or toiletries. For us, that figure is about $1,000. If that amount sounds like too much, calculate your own figure.

Keep an assortment of bills in your home stash. If the power is out and stores are unable to run their registers, a nice supply of one and five dollar bills will be very handy. A roll of quarters may come in handy for tolls, the laundromat, or pay phones. Keep your money in a home safe or fireproof box along with your other important papers.

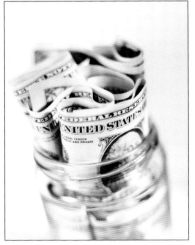

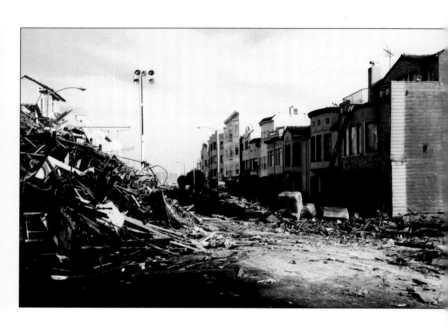

Step 2

Know the Dangers

EVERY AREA HAS ITS QUIRKS, AND MOTHER Nature is bound to surprise us from time to time with an unexpected event. It may seem an impossible task to prepare for any emergency, but the reality is that it only takes a little preplanning to understand what types of emergencies may be present in your area and the steps you need to take to be ready for them.

Earthquakes

While California is famous for its earthquakes, they can strike in any number of states. You can check with the U.S. Geological Survey (www.usgs.gov) to see if your area is prone to quakes. Even a relatively mild quake can cause injuries or service disruptions. Preparation for an earthquake begins with the basics—how to survive the quake itself. Most quake injuries are caused by falling objects, so knowing the safe zones is the key to safely getting through the tremors.

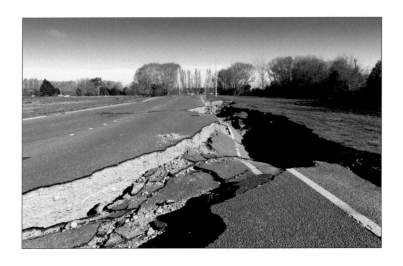

Earthquake Drill

If you are in an area that is known for earthquakes, it is essential for everyone in the family to know what to do the moment a tremor begins.

DROP down onto your hands and knees before the earth-quake knocks you down. This position protects you from falling, but still allows you to move if necessary.

COVER your head and neck (or your whole body, if possible) under the shelter of a sturdy table or desk.

HOLD ON to your shelter (or to your head and neck) until the shaking stops. Be prepared to move with your shelter if the shaking shifts it around.

At Home

Walk through the house to identify safe areas and evacuation routes.

- Review your emergency plans and supplies, checking to see if any items are missing. Replenish anything that has been used or is out of date. Make sure everyone knows where emergency lighting and other supplies are stored.

- Identify tall furniture, windows, or glass that could shatter or fall during a quake. If you are near one of these when the shaking begins, move away as quickly as possible.

- Identify tables, cabinets, or desks to use for shelter. Doorways are not adequate.

- If there is no shelter nearby, get down near an interior wall or next to low-lying furniture that won't fall on you. If you can, grab something to shield your head and face from falling objects.

- If a quake occurs during the night, stay in bed and cover your head with a pillow.

- Make sure everyone knows the location of emergency supplies.

- Mark where utility switches and turn-off valves are located.

- Discuss alternative ways to get out of the house, if damaged, and identify a safe meeting area outdoors.

- Once outside, stay away from exterior walls, utility wires, and fuel lines.

Away from Home

- Know your school's and office's emergency plans.
- Provide family members with a written emergency plan with phone numbers to carry in wallets or school bags.
- Identify a meeting place for reuniting if a quake strikes while your family is away from home.
- If you are in your car, pull over immediately, preferably away from buildings and power lines. Do not stop under an overpass. When the tremors stop, proceed with caution, watching for downed debris and damaged roads.
- If you are in a public area, do not try to rush out of the building or use elevators. Just hold on until the shaking stops, and proceed calmly to the nearest exit.

Tornado

If you live in tornado-prone area, learn about the conditions that spawn tornadoes. A simple thunderstorm can quickly cause conditions that are right for forming tornado activity, leading authorities to issue a tornado watch. Tornadoes often strike suddenly, sometimes without a thunderstorm in the vicinity. Just because you don't see a funnel cloud doesn't mean one is not lurking nearby.

When weather conditions change, stay tuned to local weather information. Take cover if you see a dark or green-colored sky, a dark, low-lying cloud, or hail. A loud roar that sounds like a freight train may accompany the approach of a funnel cloud.

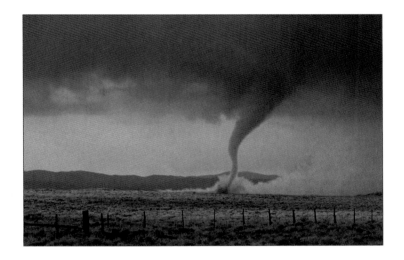

- Before storm season, review your emergency plans and supplies, checking to see if any items are missing. Replenish anything that has been used or is out of date, including batteries, water, and first aid supplies.
- If a tornado takes dead aim at your house, there is very little that can be done to prepare it for a hit. If you know ahead of time that there is a threat of severe weather, secure or put away anything that could become a flying projectile.
- Know your area's emergency warning system. If a tornado warning is issued, take cover immediately.
- If possible, go to the interior part of a basement. If you don't have a basement, go to an interior room or hallway on the lowest floor. Stay away from windows.

- Do not stay in a mobile home during a tornado warning. If you cannot get to a secure building, lie flat in a ditch or low spot on the ground.
- If you see a tornado when you are driving your car, get out immediately and seek other shelter.

After the Storm

If your home suffers damage from a tornado or severe thunderstorm:

- Check utilities and turn off gas or electricity lines until they can be inspected for damage. If you smell gas, leave the house immediately.
- Half of all injuries associated with tornadoes occur after the storms are over. Be careful of downed trees, power lines, and scattered debris. Never touch downed lines or frayed wires.
- Wear sturdy shoes, and watch for broken glass and exposed nails.
- Continue to monitor weather reports and emergency messages.
- Retrieve your insurance documents, photographed household inventory, and vehicle registration so that you will be prepared to quickly file claims.

Hurricane

If you live in hurricane country, chances are you already know the drill. The good news about hurricanes is that there is usually plenty of warning. Sky watchers track hurricanes from the

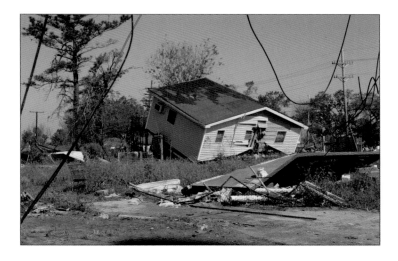

moment they form and generally have a pretty good idea where they are going. The bad news is that hurricanes can be very fickle, spinning off all sorts of weather. When a hurricane comes by, be prepared for high winds and heavy rain along with funnel cloud activity.

Because you have had the good sense to prepare, you will not be out there fighting the crowds for the last piece of plywood or gallon of water. Your stockpile is in place, and you are ready.

Do a last-minute check to make sure everything is in place. Before storm season, review your emergency plans and supplies, checking to see if any items are missing. Replenish anything that has been used or is out of date.

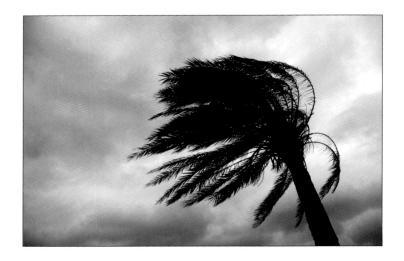

As soon as a hurricane watch is issued, you should:
- Tune in for weather updates.
- Secure or put away items such as outdoor furniture, bicycles, grills, and propane tanks.
- Cover windows and doors with plywood or boards. Ideally, you should have purchased and labeled these boards *before* hurricane season. If you can afford it, consider installing hurricane shutters.
- Plan ahead for the care of animals and pets. Emergency shelters cannot accept animals, so if possible, plan to stay with friends who can accept them or identify hotels on your evacuation route that accept animals.
- Place vehicles under cover.

- Even though you have stored water, fill sinks and bathtubs with water for an extra supply.
- Turn the thermostat on refrigerators and freezers to the coldest setting. If a freezer is only partially full, add jugs of water to fill the space. When the jugs freeze, they will help to keep your food cold longer.
- Identify the safest place to take shelter in your home. Choose an interior room without windows, such as a bathroom, and cover yourself with plywood or a mattress.
- Make sure cars have a full tank of gas. If evacuation becomes necessary, long lines quickly form and fuel may become scarce. Make sure your emergency kit is up to date and in the car. Know your evacuation route.

After the Hurricane

You may face wind and water damage after a hurricane passes. Standing water poses all sorts of risks, so don't wade through it without good boots. Snakes and stray animals may be displaced during a storm, and mosquitoes may be a problem. Don't drive through high water.

- Inspect your home for damage. Check for gas leaks and leave the house immediately if you smell gas.
- Wear waterproof boots when wading through storm water. Chances are good that it contains sewage and other runoff chemicals.
- Make sure tetanus shots are up to date. Cover hands with gloves to avoid exposure to contaminated water and accidental skin wounds.

- Listen for public announcements about the water supply. In the event of a "boil water" advisory, do not drink tap water or use it to brush your teeth unless you have boiled it for at least one full minute. You may also treat water by adding one-fourth teaspoon of bleach to a gallon of cloudy water. Let it stand for thirty minutes before using.

- Remove items that are soaked and cannot be cleaned and dried. Throw out mattresses, carpeting, upholstered furniture, pillows, and all paper products.

- Open all doors and windows. Turn on fans and dehumidifiers to remove moisture.

- Tackle mold with a mixture of one cup of bleach to one gallon of water. Open windows to make sure there is plenty of ventilation. Then scrub surfaces, rinse with clean water, and let dry. Wear boots, rubber gloves, and eye protection when cleaning with a strong bleach mixture. NEVER mix bleach and ammonia.

- Rinse off hard surfaces with fresh water and a little soap. Then spray down surfaces with a mild bleach mixture of one cup of bleach to five gallons of water.

Flood

"Water, water everywhere, but not a drop to drink" may be a very appropriate way to describe the aftermath of a flood. You will be dealing with contaminated water which contains sewage, chemical runoff, and debris of all types. Even tap water may be unusable; check with authorities to learn

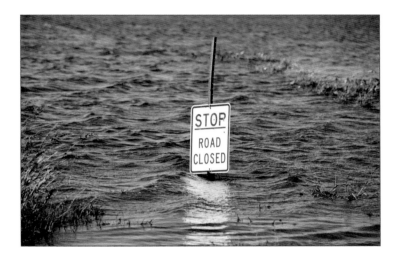

if the public water supply is safe to drink. In the event of a "boil water" advisory, do not drink tap water or use it to brush your teeth unless you have boiled it for at least one full minute. You may also treat water by adding one–fourth teaspoon of bleach to a gallon of cloudy water. Let it stand for thirty minutes before using.

- Keep children and pets out of the flood area until cleanup has been completed.
- Wear waterproof boots when wading through storm water.
- Make sure tetanus shots are up to date. Cover hands with gloves to avoid exposure to contaminated water and accidental skin wounds.

- Remove items that are soaked and cannot be cleaned and dried. Throw out mattresses, carpeting, upholstered furniture, pillows, and all paper products.
- Open all doors and windows. Turn on fans and dehumidifiers to remove moisture.
- Tackle mold with a mixture of one cup of bleach to one gallon of water. Open windows to make sure there is plenty of ventilation. Then scrub surfaces, rinse with clean water, and let dry. Wear boots, rubber gloves, and eye protection when cleaning with a strong bleach mixture. NEVER mix bleach and ammonia.
- Rinse off hard surfaces with fresh water and a little soap. Then spray down surfaces with a mild bleach mixture of one cup of bleach to five gallons of water.

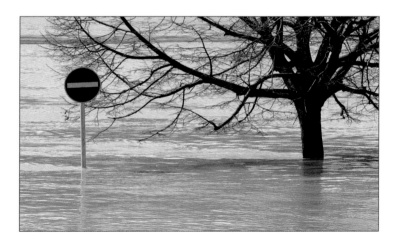

- Remove and discard drywall and insulation that has been soaked by flood waters.
- Wash clothing that has been contaminated with flood water in hot water and detergent. Go to a laundromat if possible with these clothes, until you have determined that your own water supply is clear.
- If you have to evacuate, follow posted instructions. Never drive through high, moving water.

Landslides and Mudslides

Landslides are caused by disturbances in the natural stability of a slope. They can accompany heavy rains or follow droughts and earthquakes. Mudslides develop when water-saturated rock, earth, and debris start to slip. Slides can occur anywhere there are steep slopes, particularly where there is surface run-off. Learn whether your area has ever been prone to slides like these, and prepare an emergency evacuation plan in the event of conditions that could create slides.

- Monitor weather information when there is a threat of intense storms.
- Watch for signs of increased water flow in streams and on surfaces. Tilted trees or bare spots on hill sides may indicate that the earth is shifting.
- If you hear rumbling or see rock and debris coming toward you, act quickly to move to the nearest high ground away from the path of the slide. If you can't get out, take shelter under a desk.

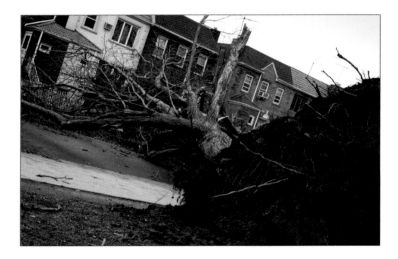

After a Slide

- Be aware that the area of the slide is very unstable. Do not inspect it on your own until all signs of additional slides have passed.
- Report damaged power wires and gas lines.
- Seek professional engineering assistance to determine the extent of the damage and alternatives.

Wildfires

Any home that is situated in a forested area needs to be prepared for the possibility of wildfire. Forest fires may start quickly under favorable wind and weather conditions and

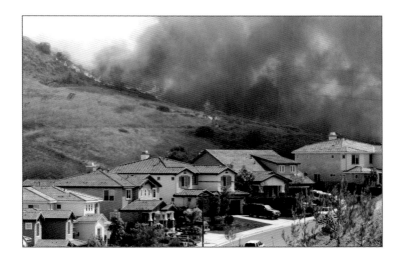

travel rapidly. But unlike weather, wildfires can be prevented, and with some preparation damage can be avoided or at least minimized.

- Know local fire laws, and only burn during approved times and conditions.
- Make certain that your driveway is clearly marked and accessible by emergency vehicles.
- Teach children about the danger of fires; keep matches and other flammable items out of their reach and make sure they know how to call for emergency assistance.
- If your home is in a forested area, create a buffer around the house to keep flames from reaching it. Make sure tree branches do not overhang the roof or chimney, and keep

dead wood pruned and removed. Clear leaves and debris away from structures and underneath porches.

- If you notice branches that could threaten power lines, call the electric company and ask for someone to come out to clear them.
- Store flammable materials, such as gas and propane, in approved containers away from the house, and make sure wood ashes are thoroughly cooled before disposing of them.
- Inside the house, make sure smoke detectors are in good working condition and fire extinguishers are up to date. Inspect and clean chimneys as needed.
- Make sure you have water outlets outside the house and a garden hose capable of reaching any area of the house.

If there is a threat of wildfire:

- Close all doors and windows.
- Shut off gas lines.
- Keep animals indoors and readily available to grab in case of evacuation.
- Wet shrubs immediately around the house, and place lawn sprinklers on the roof.
- Make sure the car is parked in a location suitable for easy escape and you have three days of emergency supplies stored inside.
- Identify escape routes and destination.

Smoke

You don't have to be in the location of a serious wildfire to be affected by it. Smoke from wildfires can hurt your eyes

Learn to Use a Fire Extinguisher

Emergency items such as fire extinguishers are only as useful as the person using them. Do an occasional check of your extinguishers to make sure there is no rust, leakage, or denting. Make sure that everyone in the family knows where extinguishers are and how to use them. Some fire departments give classes in fire extinguisher usage.

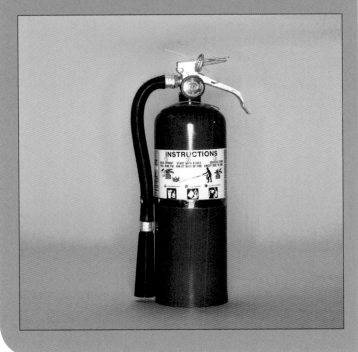

Always stand between the fire and your escape path, so that you can easily turn and run to safety. Be aware that it is not just flames that are dangerous. Smoke can overwhelm you suddenly. Know when a fire is too big to handle; the average home extinguisher only has about 10 seconds of power, so it is always safer to evacuate than try to fight a fire that is burning quickly.

OSHA makes it easy with their four-step method called PASS.

PULL the pin. This will break the seal.

AIM the nozzle at the base of the fire. Don't point it at the flames themselves. The goal is to hit the substance that is actually burning.

SQUEEZE the handle to release the extinguishing liquid.

SWEEP the fire extinguisher from side to side until extinguished.

and irritate your respiratory system. If you suffer from asthma, allergies, or other lung diseases, exposure to smoke may be very dangerous.

- Listen to public announcements on air quality and heed their directions. If you see visible smoke, take appropriate precautions.
- If you are advised to stay indoors, keep windows and doors closed. Run an air conditioner with the fresh-air intake closed. Make sure the filter is clean to prevent outdoor smoke from getting inside.

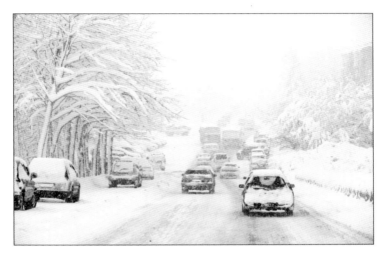

Winter Weather

Winter sports enthusiasts welcome big snowstorms as a cause for celebration. But ice storms and heavy snows can take down power lines and make for some very uncomfortable days and nights without the use of your furnace. Have a backup plan in place in case your normal source of heat is out of commission.

- Before winter, review your emergency plans and supplies, checking to see if any items are missing. Replenish anything that has been used or is out of date. Note the condition of snow shovels and other winter tools. Make sure that bags of cat litter and snow-melting salt are stored for icy conditions.
- Tune up car for cold weather and make sure winter tires are in good condition. Check your emergency car

kit and replace or replenish anything missing or out-dated.

- Winter is a particularly bad time to be low on fuel, so make sure you have at least a half a tank of gas at all times.
- Tune in for weather updates.
- If you have a fireplace, make sure you have a wood supply ready and accessible (and not under feet of snow). If you do not have a fireplace, keep one alternative heating source available. Make sure the space heater you choose is designed for indoor use. Never use generators indoors.
- Choose one room to keep warm. Arrange sleeping bags, pillows, and blankets for sleeping. If there are drafty windows or doors, put towels in place to reduce heat loss.
- Cover windows with blankets at dusk to keep out the night cold.
- Wear layered clothing to bed. Body heat escapes quickly through the head, so make sure everyone includes a hat in their nightwear.
- Make sure you have plenty of quality food and snacks so that your body can generate its own heat. Have a way to provide hot water for drinks and hot water bottles.
- Provide entertainment! Books and games are particularly welcome when you have to stay huddled in one place to stay warm.
- Keep bathroom doors open so that plumbing can be exposed to any available heat. Open cupboard doors under sinks. If possible, wrap plumbing with insulation. If you have running water, keep a little water flowing to help prevent pipes from freezing.

Radiation

A radiation emergency, such as a nuclear power plant accident or a terrorist attack, can expose people to radiation. A catastrophic release of radiation or a nuclear bomb could result in many casualties and acute radiation sickness. Immediate medical attention is required in the event of this type of exposure.

As scary as that sounds, most radiation leaks or even so-called "dirty bombs" would likely cause exposure to a relatively small amount of radiation. This level of exposure may not result in immediate sickness, although there may be cancer concerns over the long term. If you are informed of potential radiation exposure, the best place to be is at home.

- If you are outside when an alert occurs, get inside as quickly as possible. Remove your outer layer of clothing, and place it in a bag or out-of-the-way location. Wash skin that was exposed to the air with soap and water.
- If you live near a nuclear power plant, you can monitor radiation levels with a RAD sticker.
- If you are contaminated, you can spread the contamination by touching surfaces or even walking through a house. Body fluids from internally contaminated people can contaminate other people in the household.
- The safest place to be in case of radiation leaks is at home. Make sure your home is ready for "sheltering in place" and has an adequate supply of safe drinking water and food to keep you comfortable indoors for several days.

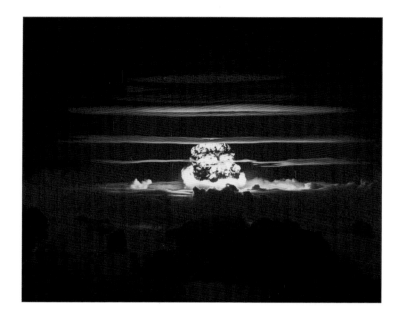

- Close and lock all doors and windows. Close fireplace dampers.
- Turn off fans, air conditioners, or heating units that bring in fresh air from outdoors.
- Move to an interior room or basement.
- Make sure you have a reliable source for news and information.
- Potassium iodide (KI) should only be taken in a radiation emergency that involves the release of radioactive iodine, such as an accident at a nuclear power plant or the explosion of a nuclear bomb. You should only take KI if you have

been instructed to do so by local public health or emergency management officials.

Evacuation

Because there is no way to see which way a radiation plume is moving, it is important to listen to the advice of local professionals before deciding to evacuate the area. If you are asked to evacuate, act quickly.

- Close up your house and turn off all heat and air conditioning.
- Follow the directions of local authorities to avoid the radiation plume.
- In the car, keep windows closed and ventilation systems off.

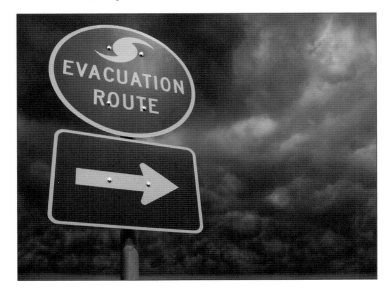

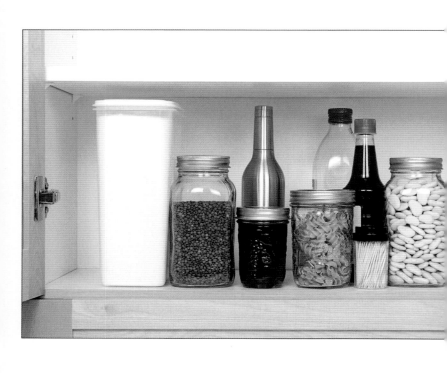

Step 3

Prepare Your Home

YOUR HOME IS YOUR REFUGE AND SHOULD BE able to shelter and protect you whatever the conditions in the outside world. Take the time TODAY to make your house a safe and secure place to shelter you in a time of crisis. The first step is to set a minimum standard for yourself—you should be able to ride out bad weather and emergency situations for at least three days, with safety measures in place, a source of alternate lighting, backup forms of energy, stockpiles of food, and plenty of water.

Organize

In this tech-friendly world, it is tempting to keep track of many of your most important accounts and policies online. But in the event of an emergency, life can get frustrating in a hurry without important contacts and policy numbers at the ready.

Buy a small home safe or fireproof box and create a comprehensive list of everything you might need to know in the event of an emergency. Your safe should contain the following:

- Records of all your account passwords
- Copies of each of your credit cards (front and back)
- All of your insurance policies, along with the contact name and number of your agent

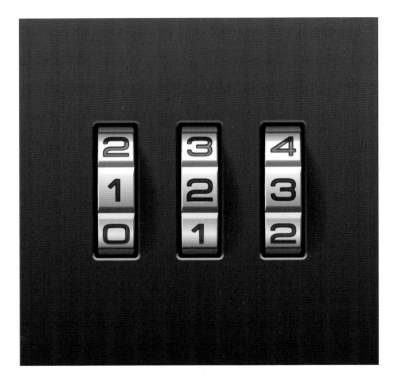

- Copy of all driver's licenses and passports
- Photo identification of children
- Animal registration, vaccination records, and photo identi-fication of your pet
- List of doctors' names, addresses, and telephone numbers
- List of all family medical prescriptions, with strength and dosage
- Birth certificates and car titles

- A list of any important valuables (keep a video record of every room in your house, as well as boats and other vehicles so that you can refer to them for insurance purposes)
- Ready cash in small denominations, including coins

Is your house ready for any emergency? Walk through your house and yard, and ask yourself the following questions:

- Are smoke detectors installed on every level of the house, and are batteries current?
- Do you have a working, wired, landline phone?
- Are battery-operated devices all in working order?
- Are mirrors and heavy pictures well-secured?
- Are hallways and other exits clear and uncluttered?
- Are bookshelves secured to the wall, with heavy items on the lowest shelves?
- Is there a fire extinguisher on each level of the house, and do you know how to use it?
- Are flammable or highly reactive chemicals such as bleach, ammonia, and paint thinners stored safely and out of the reach of children?
- Do you know how to turn off water and gas mains, and shut down electricity?
- Are sump pumps working? Are generators or other emergency devices in good working order?
- Do all doors and windows have working locks?
- Is your house number visible from the street?
- Are there any trees, limbs, utility poles, or other objects that could cause safety issues?

- Are drainage outlets, eaves troughs, and gutters clear?
- Do I have charcoal or extra propane for my outdoor grills?

Create a Home Emergency Kit

Natural disasters can cause a lot of chaos, and even with the best possible plans in place, it may take emergency personnel a few days to reach everyone and make supplies available.

So what does your family need to get by? Your emergency kit should be designed for a minimum of three days and include the following:

- Water: you will need about one gallon of water per person per day to be used for both drinking and sanitation.
- Food: you will want at least a three-day supply of non-perishable food that requires minimal or no cooking. If you have babies, make sure formula and diapers are included.
- Manual can opener
- Pet food, water, and other supplies. A leash or pet crate may be handy for keeping your pet out of harm's way.
- Battery-powered or hand-crank radio
- Flashlight
- Extra batteries
- First aid kit, along with important prescription medications. When you get new prescription glasses, add your old ones to the kit.
- An extra set of car keys
- Emergency shelter, including plastic sheeting or tarps and duct tape to repair walls or create a shelter in place
- Moist towelettes and garbage bags for personal sanitation

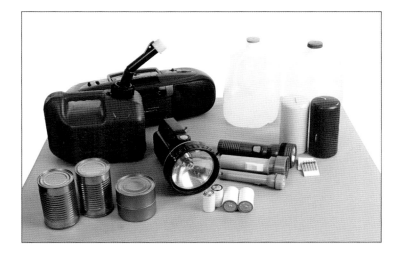

- A basic tool kit, including a hammer, screwdriver, wrench, and utility knife
- Local maps
- Cell phone with home and car charger or solar charger
- Sleeping bag or warm blanket for each person
- Complete change of clothing, including a long sleeved shirt, long pants, and sturdy shoes
- Household chlorine bleach and medicine dropper when diluted, nine parts water to one part bleach, bleach can be used as a disinfectant.
- Spare tank of propane for outdoor cooking
- Fire extinguisher
- Matches and candles in a waterproof container

• Paper and pencil, and a supply of books, games, playing cards, or puzzles

Choose a cool, dry location to store your emergency supplies. Label food items with the date you are placing them in storage. Keep food in tightly closed plastic containers to keep out rodents, insects, and excess moisture. Place sleeping bags and spare clothing in plastic garbage bags. Tools and other gear can be stored together in another large plastic container. We use five-gallon plastic buckets for all our supplies.

Maintain your supplies by refreshing them every six months or so. Check dates and discard old items. Label water containers and replace drinking water with fresh containers. Think about any new or different needs and add to your kit accordingly.

The Seventy-Two-Hour Plan

The reality is that the most common emergencies last just three days or less. Bad weather is the most common cause for short-term emergency planning. Whether you are interested in long-

Are your pets ready for an emergency?

One of the most heartbreaking sights of Hurricane Katrina was the faces of lost and stranded animals. When disaster strikes, it may feel like all you can do to get yourself ready, but the animals in your life are counting on you for protection, so take a little time to get them ready too.

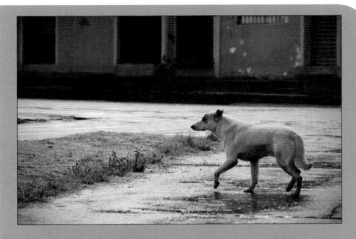

- Place a rescue alert sticker on the window of your home so emergency workers know that animals may be inside the house.
- Make sure your pet's collar has current address tags and updated immunization tags. Even better, have your vet microchip your animal. Most animal shelters can scan for microchips, so pets can be identified even if they lose their collars.
- Have a bug-out pack ready for pets, with a leash and an extra collar, three to seven days worth of food and water, feeding bowl, blanket, and crate.
- Photocopy veterinary and immunization records; if you have to shelter the dog in a kennel you will need to

provide evidence of health. Include photographs of
pets in case they get lost.

- Arrange for a safe shelter for your pet in the event that
you have to leave them behind. Locate recommended
kennels in other cities, arrange with a friend or family member who can take pets, and know what hotels
will accept pets.

- Keep a leash near the door at all times in case you
need to make a hasty exit. If there is a threat of bad
weather, make sure to keep pets in the house. Bad
weather can upset pets, and they may be hard to locate
or even run off if they become disoriented.

term self-sufficiency or not, everyone should have a plan that
will allow them to get through three days off the grid in relative
comfort.

Water

You should always have at least one gallon of potable water per
person in your household per day for at least three days. An
additional gallon per day should also be on hand for personal
hygiene and basic cleaning. For a couple with two children,
that is 12 gallons for drinking and 12 more for other uses. Keep
gallon-size jugs for drinking, and use five-gallon buckets to
store your personal hygiene water.

Food

Your food plan should include the following for *each person* in your household:

- Grains: a minimum of eighteen servings of grains, breads, rice, or pasta (at least six servings per day per person)
- Fruit: a minimum of six servings of any type of fruit, avocados, or tomatoes (at least two servings per day per person)
- Vegetables: a minimum of nine servings of any type of vegetable (at least three servings per day per person)
- Protein: a minimum of six servings of any type of meat, legumes, eggs, peanut butter, or nuts (at least two servings per day per person)

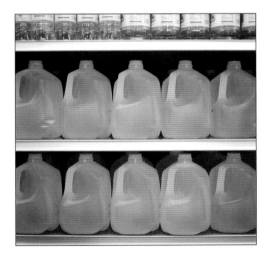

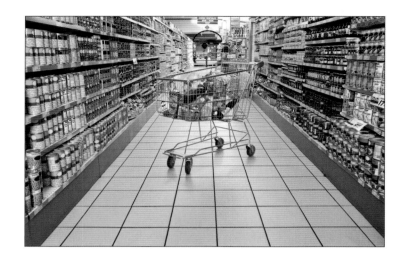

- Dairy: a minimum of six servings of milk, yogurt, or cheese (at least two servings per day per person)

A three day emergency menu might look something like this:

Day 1

Breakfast
Granola with milk and canned peaches

Lunch
Split pea soup
Cornbread

Daily Servings

Low	Moderate	High
Sedentary Women	Most Children *	Teen Boys
Older Adults	Teen Girls	Many Active Men
	Active Women	Very Active Women
	Pregnant Women	
	Nursing Women	
	Sedentary Men	
Calories		
1,600	2,200	2,800
Water		
1 gallon	1 gallon	1 gallon
Grains		
6	9	11
Vegetables		
3	4	5
Fruit		
2	3	4
Dairy		
2-3	2-4	2-5
Meat		
2	2	2

Dinner
Angel hair pasta with spaghetti sauce, white beans, and spinach

<u>Day 2</u>

Breakfast
Oatmeal with brown sugar, nuts, raisins, and milk

Lunch
Tuna salad with brown bread

Dinner
Rice
Refried black beans
Corn

<u>Day 3</u>

Breakfast
Pancakes with syrup
Stewed apples

Lunch
Tomato soup
Cheese and rye crackers

Dinner
Brown rice and lentils
Canned peas

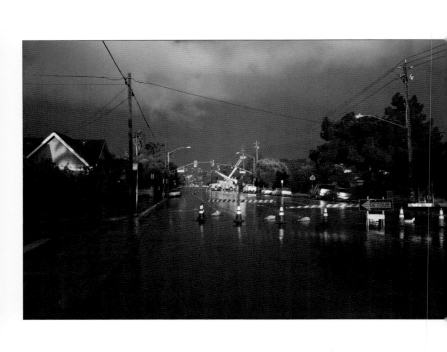

Step 4

Plan for Losing Power

CREATE A PLAN SO THAT LOSING POWER DOES not constitute an emergency. It is as simple as knowing how your house works. If you don't understand how your various systems function, find an expert to walk you through it and explain.

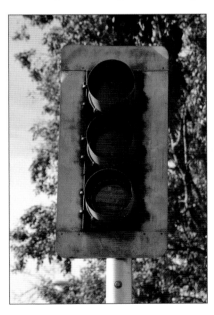

- If you have appliances, a sump pump, or medical devices that are absolutely dependent on power, have a backup generator in place.

- If you are on city water, you will probably still have access, but your hot water heater may not work. Even gas heaters often have electrical ignitions, so double-check. If the power is off for a while, your municipal system may have purification problems and send out a "MUST BOIL" alert to customers.

- If you have your own well, you will not have water because your pump requires electricity.

- If you use a well and have very inefficient toilets, you will need a LOT more water for flushing. Replace these with high efficiency toilets that only require a gallon of water for flushing.

- Know how your heating system or furnace works. Furnaces have ignitions and blower systems that require electricity, so they will not be a source for heat in a power outage.

- Do your pipes rely on heat tape to prevent freezing? If so, you might want to think about wrapping them with some other type of insulation.

- If you have a security system, make sure the backup battery is charged.

- Place high-quality surge protectors on all your electronic devices and computers. Back up computer files regularly.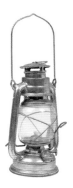

- Have a backup plan for charging phones and laptops. Car chargers or small solar chargers will come in handy for keeping things useable.

- If you have electric garage door openers, know how to open the door manually.

- How many other items that you rely on run on electricity? We were annoyed to realize that our electric leaf blowers were unusable when a storm took out our power, so we couldn't do as much cleanup as we wanted. We got a gas-powered version soon after.

- If you have canned food, make sure you have a manual can opener.
- If you want to use candles for lighting, make sure that you have a lantern for keeping flames enclosed. Do not burn anything with an exposed flame.
- Dark feels even darker when the power goes out. Consider installing solar-powered path lighting to give you a greater feeling of security.

Lights-Out Kit

Be able to quickly put your hands on your lights-out kit so you don't have to go fumbling around for it after dark. We keep our kit near the bed so that we can grab it in the middle of the night, if necessary. Even if it's still daylight when the power goes out, get your kit out and place it where it is readily accessible to everyone in the family.

Your kit should include:
- One flashlight with batteries for every family member
- One larger fluorescent lantern for illuminating a whole room
- An LED headlamp, useful for hands-free damage assessment and repairs
- Battery-operated radio and clock

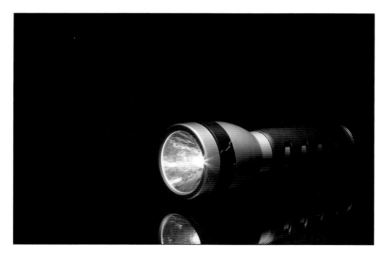

- Extra batteries
- A cooler and ice for items you will need easy access to, like baby formula or refrigerated medicine
- A basic tool kit
- A car charger or solar charger
- A list of important phone numbers

In addition, if there is a threat of a storm:
- Make sure you have propane for emergency stoves
- Make sure you have gasoline for your chainsaw
- Make sure there is cash in your wallet
- Always have at least half a tank of gas in the car
- Turn the refrigerator and freezer to the highest setting

Entertaining Yourself without Power

I once heard someone refer to the loss of electricity as being like a death in the family. And it is true. There is something about the familiar buzz of accessible power that is reassuring us. Interaction with the outside world and entertainment of all types is at your fingertips. For some people, this loss is the greatest discomfort of all.

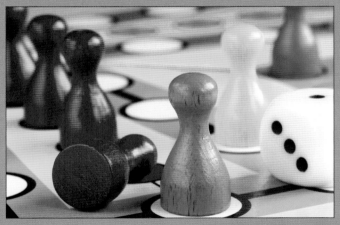

So how do you plan to entertain yourself if the power goes out?

Board Games. You kind of forgot about them, didn't you? But these old reliables are still fun and can be a source of several hours of amusement. Stock Monopoly, Scrabble, Yahtzee, and Risk for the older members of the family. Keep Candyland, Parcheesi, and checkers for the younger set.

Cards. Whether it's poker for a crowd or solitaire for one, a deck of cards can help you while away several hours. A rousing game of poker while sitting in the dark of a hurricane strengthens the will and keeps up the spirits.

Books. You might love that e-reader, but batteries don't last forever, so keep a handful of your favorite books in your emergency gear. Choose adventure stories that children and adults enjoy, and read aloud from the latest Harry Potter or the Hunger Games series.

Art and Imagination. Release your creativity and create plays, pantomimes, and story telling contests. Keep art supplies available for the kids for drawing and coloring.

Digital Entertainment. Okay, so you really are dependent on that tech fix? Tablets, portable DVD players, and handheld electronic games may help the time go by. Just make sure to have plenty of batteries and alternate charging devices.

A Glass of Wine. Sometimes you just have to take a break from surviving and have a glass of wine. Here's a highly efficient, low-energy way to chill a bottle of white wine in less than six minutes: stand your wine bottle in an ice bucket and surround it with ice. Sprinkle on a handful of salt and a cup of water. The salt breaks down the ice, which will make the wine cold faster. Keep it nearby and give the bottle a spin every now and then to make it chill even faster. Be careful though, low lighting and warm fireplaces combined with wine has been known to produce children. (There are many examples of blizzard-induced baby booms!) Make sure you have also stored adequate contraception, just in case.

Powerless Eating

Consider what your family would eat if no cooking sources were available for a few days. I keep canned brown bread, as well as a supply of high-energy snacks such as nuts, peanut butter, crackers, protein bars, and GORP handy. It also helps to have a few treats on hand, such as candy, pudding cups, or cocoa mix.

Another way to plan for this type of short-term emergency is by purchasing precooked and packaged meals that have been freeze-dried or dehydrated. You can choose military-grade MREs (that's Meals Ready to Eat) that can be kept in storage for up to five years, or you can

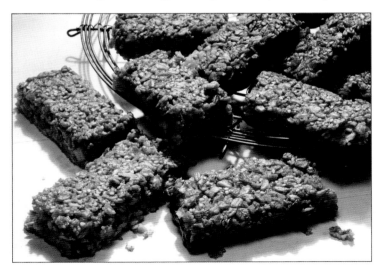

opt for an assortment of basic food stuffs that will last as long as twenty-five years.

Refrigerated Food

Refrigerated food is good for only a few hours after the power goes out. Any food requiring refrigeration that is held above 40°F for more than two hours is considered dangerous. If a major power outage lasts more than about four hours, it is likely that most of your refrigerated food will have to be discarded. There are a few exceptions, like hard cheeses and some fresh produce. See the chart below to determine what can be salvaged.

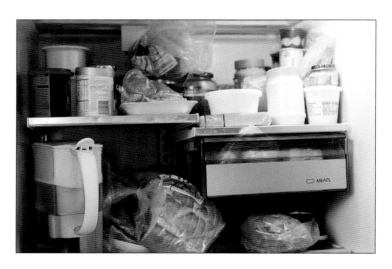

REFRIGERATED FOODS – KEEP OR DISCARD?

DISCARD	KEEP
MEATS AND PROTEINS	
Raw or leftover cooked meat, poultry, fish, or seafood	Hard cheeses: cheddar, swiss, provolone
Soy meat substitutes, tofu	Processed cheeses
Thawing meat or poultry	Parmesan, romano, whole or grated
Meat, tuna, shrimp, chicken, or egg salads	Butter, margarine
Gravy, stuffing, broth	
Lunchmeats, hot dogs, bacon, sausage, dried beef	
Canned hams labeled "Keep refrigerated"	
Canned meats and fish, opened	
Casseroles, soups, stews	
DAIRY	
Soft cheeses	
Shredded cheeses	
Low-fat cheeses	
Milk and milk products	
Baby formula, opened	
Fresh eggs, eggs hard-cooked in shell, egg dishes, egg products	
Custards, puddings, quiche	

Continued

DISCARD	KEEP
FRUITS	
Fresh fruits, cut	Fruit juices, opened
	Canned fruits, opened
	Fresh fruits, coconut, raisins, dried fruits, candied fruits, dates
SAUCES AND CONDIMENTS	
Fish sauces, oyster sauce	Worcestershire, soy, barbecue, and hoisin sauces
Opened mayonnaise, tartar sauce, horseradish	Fish sauces, oyster sauce Opened vinegar-based dressings
Opened cream-based dressings	
Spaghetti sauce, opened	
PACKAGED PRODUCTS	
Refrigerated biscuits, rolls, cookie dough	Bread, rolls, cakes, muffins, quick breads, tortillas
Cooked pasta, rice, potatoes	Peanut butter
Pasta salads with mayonnaise or vinaigrette	Jelly, relish, taco sauce, mustard, catsup, olives, pickles
Fresh pasta Cheesecake	Breakfast foods—waffles, pancakes, bagels
Pastries, cream filled	Pies, fruit
Pies—custard, cheese filled, or chiffon; quiche	

Continued

DISCARD	KEEP
Greens, precut, prewashed, packaged	Fresh mushrooms, herbs, spices
Vegetables, cooked	Vegetables, raw
Vegetable juice, opened	
Baked potatoes	
Commercial garlic in oil	
LEFTOVERS	
Potato salad	Fresh pasta
Casseroles, soups, stews	
Pizza, any topping	

Frozen Food

Freezing is an easy and convenient way to preserve meat and homegrown produce. It is also very good for retaining the nutritional value of your food. The problem is that this storehouse of surplus food is dependent on the power staying on.

Food in the freezer will generally keep two to three days after the power goes out. There are a handful of things you can do to keep the cold in as long as possible:

- Choose a chest freezer over an upright one. Chest freezers retain their temperature longer.
- Avoid opening the freezer door unless absolutely necessary.
- Sort meats on one side of the freezer and other foods on the other side. That way, juices from meat products won't contaminate other foods. If you are expecting an outage,

stack foods on top of one another to help them stay frozen longer.

- Don't run a half-empty freezer. It is inefficient, and the food will melt even faster. If you have a lot of spare space in your freezer, fill milk or soda containers with water and place them in the freezer along with your other items. (Make sure to leave space in the bottles—water expands when frozen.) The extra ice will keep frozen foods cold longer. The other advantage is that this stored water provides another source for emergency drinking water.
- Thawed food should be used as soon as possible.

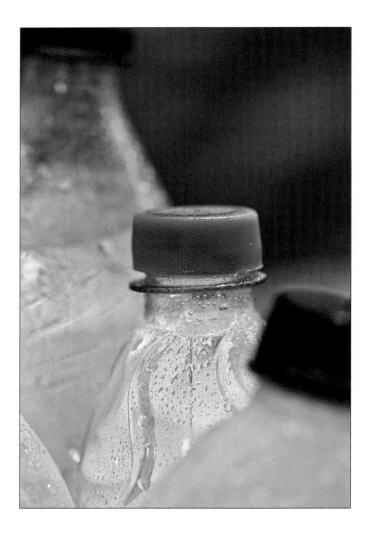

Step 5

Store Water

WATER IS THE MOST CRITICAL ELEMENT OF survival. In spite of the discomfort hunger can cause, the reality is that most of us could get by days and even weeks without food. But we can't last a week without water. In fact, the average person in a reasonably comfortable environment, using very little energy, could probably only survive three to five days without water.

How much water do you need?

Something as simple as an electrical outage can throw your normal routine into a tailspin. Suddenly your pump won't work, making that tap water just outside your grasp. For this reason, you should always have at least a three-day supply of potable drinking water for every person and animal in the household. For adults and large dogs, that's about a gallon a day. Children and small pets may be able to get by with a little less. That means that for a family of four, you should always have at least twelve gallons of drinking water available. For cleaning and hygiene, another gallon per person per day would also be desirable.

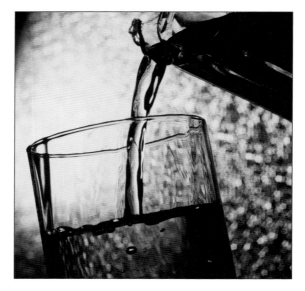

Floods and storms can damage or contaminate wells and municipal water systems, potentially making access to previously–available resources out of the question for longer periods of time. Water is very heavy, which makes keeping a three-month supply rather daunting. That's ninety gallons per person, *just for drinking*. Plan on another gallon per day for sanitation and personal needs.

Storing Water

Tap water is safe to store, so filling your own food–grade containers is a good way to get started. For large quantities of water, consider water storage barrels that can contain up to fifty-five-gallons—enough for about a month for two people. Fifty-five-gallon food-quality drums are relatively easy to fill and store, but when full weigh over 400 pounds. We prefer to store smaller containers, including five-gallon drums. Packaged water is available in every size imaginable, from personal bottle size to sealed five-gallon containers, and many of these can be reused for water storage.

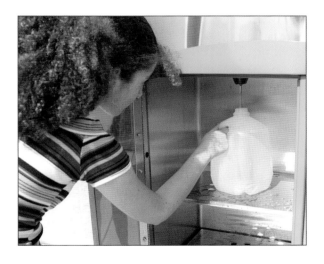

Keep water in a cool, dark place. Though freezing will not hurt water, it could cause overfilled containers to leak. Water does not have a definite shelf life, but it doesn't hurt to check large containers for cloudiness before use. Sealed containers should stay fresh indefinitely.

If your freezer is not full, consider keeping containers of water in there too. Frozen water containers will help keep the freezer cold longer, and provide an extra source of water as they melt. Just make sure to leave headroom for expansion in the water containers you store there.

Purifying Nonpotable Water

Water that has not been treated could contain organisms that may cause serious gastric distress. Water from lakes or streams, or rainwater in your outdoor rain barrels should always be treated before use. This applies to drinking water, as well as any water that you use to clean food, wash dishes, or brush your teeth.

If water is cloudy or contains particulates, strain it before disinfecting. Home water filters are not designed for disinfecting water but they may help to make your disinfected water more palatable, so it's a good idea to run water through your filter after boiling or bleaching it.

Boiling

Bring water to a full rolling boil and continue for three to five minutes. Cool and store.

If you want to keep sterilized water available for special purposes, such as infant formula or sterile wound cleaning, you may boil water and then process glass jars of your sterilized water in a water bath canner.

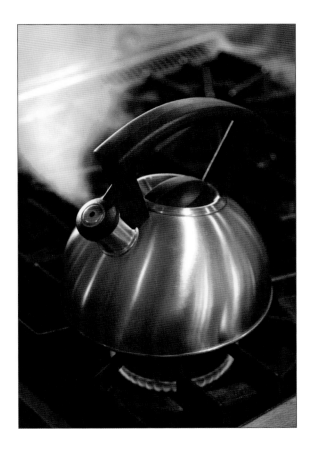

Clean and sterilize quart jars, and fill with your boiled water, leaving about an inch of headspace. Tighten lids and rings into place and process for about twenty-five minutes.

Disinfecting with Bleach

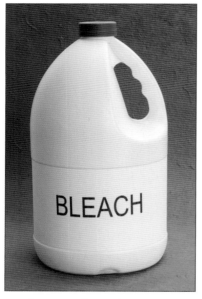

You can make water safe to drink by adding bleach. Bleach by itself is pretty toxic, so it is important to follow the instructions for purifying water exactly. Use only a pure liquid bleach, not one that contains soap or any other ingredients. The label should say "Sodium Hypochlorite." Most household bleaches come in a concentration of about 5-6 percent. To purify one gallon of water, add one-eighth teaspoon of bleach. For five gallons, use one-half teaspoon. Shake the container to thoroughly incorporate the bleach into the water. Let your treated water sit for at least forty-five minutes before using to kill any bacteria that may be present.

Got Bleach?

The surprising thing about bleach is not how useful it is, but how little is actually needed to do the job.

- Place one-half teaspoon (yes, that's all) into five gallons of water to purify it for drinking. If the water is cloudy, use twice that amount.
- Bleach is indispensable for removing mold and mildew. One cup of bleach in two gallons of water will remove stains from hard surfaces. Scrub, rinse, and repeat if necessary.
- Bleach makes a great disinfectant. Just mix one table-spoon of bleach in a gallon of water to clean almost anything.
- Sanitize secondhand items, old dishes, and glassware by soaking in one gallon of dishwater with a couple of tablespoons of bleach. Ten minutes should do the trick. Rinse and air dry items in the sun.
- One-fourth teaspoon of bleach in a quart of water will keep cut flowers fresh longer.

Water for Hygiene

In addition to drinking water, you will want an available source of water for cleaning, maintaining your toilet, and basic hygiene. When there is a threat of storms, simply filling the bathtub may give you the extra water you need for these basic tasks. Like-wise, outdoor rain barrels are great for collecting this type of emergency water. Swimming pool or hot tub water may be handy for NONdrinking purposes, like cleaning or flushing toilets, but because of the chemicals used in this type of water,

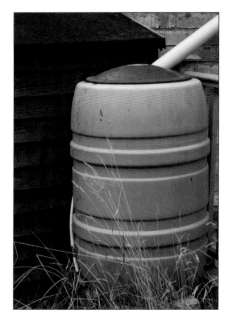

avoid it as a source of drinking water.

Running Your Toilet

There are two ways to use your toilet during a power outage. The first is to fill the toilet tank with water and flush as usual. The second way is simpler: just pour water directly into the bowl after use to flush waste. Make sure to keep some water in the bowl at all times so fumes from the sewer or septic tank don't seep into the house. Only flush when absolutely necessary!

If you don't have enough water for running your toilet, there are camping toilets and even disposable bucket toilets designed for camping.

Laundry

Faced with days without power, you may wonder what happens the day you run out of clean clothes. Hot water, a washtub, and a scrubber will accomplish the task, along with a heavy-duty clothesline. But a little forethought can keep the laundry from piling up.

For clothes that are not actually dirty, rather than tossing them in the laundry basket as you normally would, spray a little fabric freshener on them and hang them out in a well-ventilated place at the end of the day. Consider adding a T-shirt under your other clothes; this underlayer can be washed more easily than a heavy sweatshirt. Keep certain clothes for messy tasks like cooking, and change into those before you get started. If you do get a stain, stop and treat it immediately rather than changing clothes completely. A pen-style laundry stain remover can rescue a shirt for another day of use.

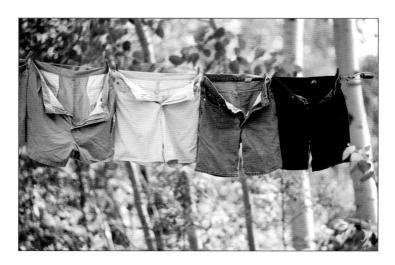

Personal Hygiene

Days without a shower can seem like torture for those of us accustomed to this everyday luxury. As long as you have enough water available, you can fashion a bath of sorts from hot water and soap. We keep wet wipes in our storage specifically for power outages. Not only does this save a lot of water, we find that using them for everything from washing faces and hands to substituting them for toilet paper keeps everyone feeling (relatively) fresh. Likewise, a squirt of liquid hand sanitizer allows you to avoid reaching for the water bottle unless you have something on your hands that really requires rinsing. A spray bottle of water can also go a long way after a hot or sweaty day.

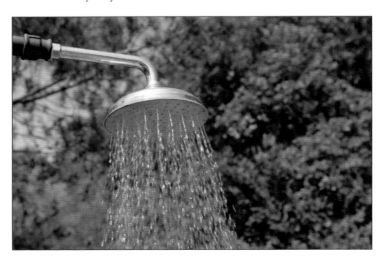

Of course, nothing beats a good shower! We discovered the solar shower years ago when we started camping. This simple five-gallon PVC bag hangs in the sun where it can warm up water, and comes with a small shower head.

Conserving Water

The first step to having enough water is knowing how to use it. We learned this the hard way one year when a particularly bad drought threatened our water supplies for several months. We learned in a hurry when and how to make the most of our water supply, how to find alternatives to running water, and how to collect and store water. We quickly replaced our high-flow toilets with more efficient models and learned to stay clean with a minimum of showers. Paper plates and utensils were a lifesaver.

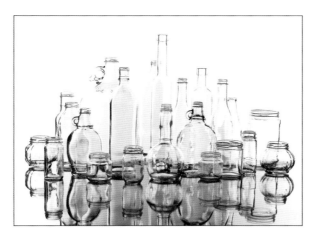

Before you have a water crisis, conduct an audit of your house to make sure you are doing all you can to conserve:

- Check faucets, pipes, and toilets for leaks.
- Install water-saving showerheads and toilets.
- Run the laundry and dishwasher only when you have a full load.
- Learn to take shorter showers, and shut off water while you brush your teeth or shave.
- Keep a bottle of cold water in the refrigerator rather than running tap water until it is cold.
- Outside, mulch plants to keep the soil around them moist.
- Add rain barrels or a rainwater tank to catch runoff.

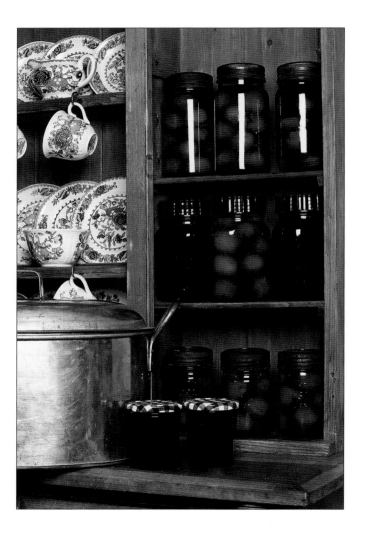

Step 6
Fill Your Pantry

A LONG-TERM FOOD STORAGE PLAN IS YOUR very own "food bank account." You want that bank account to be a sound investment, one that you have ready access to, and one that will provide you exactly what you need when you need it. Remember: no matter what a great deal it is, how long its shelf life, or how practical it might sound, there is absolutely no point in storing food you don't want to eat.

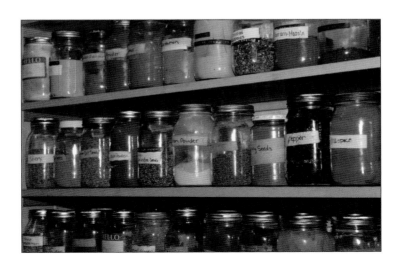

So what should go into your food pantry?

Build your own individualized food pantry using the common-sense "eat what you store, store what you eat" approach. This means that you only buy food you actually want to eat, food that your family is accustomed to, and food that you actually use every day, rather than accumulating food and locking it up tight for some future imagined time.

Because you are always rotating through your pantry, you don't have to wait for a full-scale emergency to use your food. You always have your own piggy bank to draw from, even when it's just a week where your budget is a little pinched.

To start creating your own customized food pantry, consider the kinds of meals your family currently eats. Look at your favorite recipes and see how you might adapt those to items that are in a storage pantry. Try to take a balanced approach to meal planning and storage. The following ratios are an example of foods that would contribute to a balanced diet:

> **PROTEIN:** 13 percent of your food supply. This category includes legumes, meat, peanut butter, and assorted nuts.
>
> **GRAINS:** 40 percent of your food supply. This would include cereals like oatmeal, as well as pasta, rice, and breads.
>
> **VEGETABLES:** 20 percent of your food supply. This would include carrots, peas, green beans, corn, and other vegetables.
>
> **DAIRY:** 12 percent of your food supply. This would include milk, yogurt, and cheeses.

FRUITS: 15 percent of your food supply. This would include canned peaches, berries, and other fruits, including tomatoes.

These ratios are only a guideline and apply to a full day, so you may find that more cereal and fruit are eaten at breakfast, while proteins and vegetables make up the rest of the day's meals.

Staples

Your long-term food storage plan begins with the fundamentals, including grains, beans, fats, sweeteners, dairy items, and basic baking ingredients.

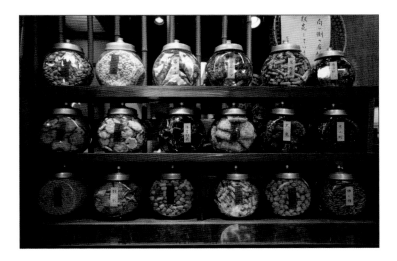

At the most basic level, every person needs about one pound of dry matter every day to survive. Dry matter may mean legumes, grains, sugar, pasta, dried vegetables, or rice. This dry matter represents calories, the stuff that is needed to produce energy in the body. A pound of dry matter represents about 1,600 calories, a reasonable amount of energy for the average adult. A consistent diet of dry matter would, of course, be deadly dull, and over the course of a few months, the body would begin to suffer from the lack of protein, fresh greens, and essential vitamins. Still, it is good to keep in mind as you make decisions about what to store.

Some people do keep an emergency pantry that contains only these essentials—whole grains, dried beans, oils, and sweeteners. The problem is that these foods require that you to cook in a way that may not be compatible with your current lifestyle. You need to have a basic understanding of cooking and baking techniques, as well as a high tolerance for boring meals! If you decide to make these staples the center of your food pantry, take the time to learn to use them in your everyday meals.

A One-Year Emergency Pantry

To feed a family of four for a full year, a pantry that consisted entirely of staple ingredients would look something like this:

500 pounds of whole grain wheat for grinding	100 pounds of cornmeal
	100 pounds of oats
100 pounds of flour	50 pounds of quinoa

50 pounds of millet
200 pounds of rice
100 pounds of pasta
120 pounds of dried beans
20 pounds of lentils
20 pounds of split peas
40 pounds of soy beans
16 pounds of peanut butter
1½ gallons of dehydrated eggs
50 pounds of TVP
160 pounds of sugar
12 pounds of honey
12 pounds of molasses or
    maple syrup

12 pounds of jam
12 pounds of sprouting seeds
40 quarts of vegetable oil
240 pounds of dry milk
48 cans of evaporated milk
4 pounds of baking powder
4 pounds of baking soda
2 pounds of yeast
20 pounds of salt
2 gallons of vinegar
20 pounds of dry soup mix
A variety of spices and
    seasonings

Long-Term Food Storage

Every item in your storage pantry wants three conditions to maintain its optimum quality: cool, dry, and dark. High temperatures, humid or wet conditions, and exposure to light are the primary causes of spoiled food. In addition, food must be kept safe from bugs and rodents. Keep these factors in mind when storing any food products. The following are specific recommendations for each food group.

Whole grains, dried beans, and white rice are very durable, but they prefer to be stored in a cool, dry location. Flours, sugars, oils, dry milk, and canned goods want the same conditions, but generally have a shorter shelf life, so check on life expectancy before deciding on how much to store. Temperatures of 50–60°F are ideal for ensuring maximum longevity. Overheating or wide temperature swings will shorten shelf life. Likewise, humidity causes challenges. Any time moisture is present there is a danger for molds and bacteria to grow.

SHELF LIFE OF FOODS

"Sealed" refers to hermetically sealed containers. These are estimates, and will vary based on storage conditions. Check the manufacturer's dates for specific information.

For commercial products, check the manufacturer's "best by" date, and use that as your "sealed" date.

PROTEINS	SEALED	OPEN
Canned ham	2-5 years	3-4 days in refrigerator
Freeze-dried meats	25 years	1 year
Commercially made jerky	2 years	1 year
Home-dried jerky	1–2 months	1–2 months
Hard/dry sausage	6 weeks in pantry	3 weeks in refrigerator
Dried eggs	12-15 months	Refrigerate after opening. Use within 7 to 10 days. Use reconstituted egg mix immediately or refrigerate and use within 1 hour.
Canned tuna	18 months	3-4 days in refrigerator
Other canned meats	18 months	3-4 days in refrigerator

LEGUMES	SEALED	OPEN
Dried beans	30 years	5 years
Instant dried beans	30 years	1 year
TVP	10 years	1 year
Peanuts		
Peanut butter, natural	2 years from manufacturer's date	2–3 months
Peanut butter, emulsified	2 years from manufacturer's date	18 months
Peanut butter powder	4 years	1 year

GRAINS AND FLOUR

Wheat	10–12 years	2 years
Dry corn	10–12 years	3 years
Millet	10–12 years	4 years
Flax	10–12 years	4 years
Barley	8 years	18 months
Quinoa	20 years	1 year
Rolled oats	8 years	1 year
Whole wheat flour	2 years	6 months
White flour	4 years	1 year
Spelt flour	5 years	8–12 months
Flaxseed flour	1 year	2–3 months
White rice	10 years	1 year
Brown and wild rice	1–2 years	6 months
Pasta	8 years	3 years

Continued

NUTS	SEALED	OPEN
In the shell	9 months	6 months
Shelled	2 years	18 months

FRUITS AND VEGETABLES

Low-acid canned goods, such as soups, vegetables, stews	2-5 years	3-4 days in refrigerator
High-acid canned goods, such as fruits, tomatoes, and vinegar-based items	12-18 months	5-7 days in refrigerator
Home-canned foods	1 year	3-4 days in refrigerator
Dehydrated fruit	25 years	12-18 months
Dehydrated vegetables	25 years	1-2 years

BAKING SUPPLIES

Yeast	2 years	4 months
Honey	10 years	2 years
White sugar	30 years	2 years
Brown sugar	10 years	1 year
Molasses	2 years	6 months
Baking powder, baking soda, and salt	30 years	2 years
Vinegar	2 years	1 year
Spices and seasonings	2 years	2 years
Boullion	5 years	2 years

OILS	SEALED	OPEN
Cooking oils	6 months	3-6 months
Shortening	2 years from manufac-tured date	1 year
Shortening powder	10 years	1 year
DAIRY PRODUCTS		
Dry milk	25 years	2 years
Sour cream powder	10 years	1 year
Cheese, dried	15 years	6 months
Butter powder	5 years	9 months
OTHER		
Seeds for sprouting	5 years	4 years

All bulk foods used for long-term storage should be carefully sealed to keep them safe from pests and rodents. To store a large quantity of dried bulk foods, choose food-grade five-gallon buckets with gasket lids. Line each bucket with a Mylar bag. Place one 500cc oxygen absorber in the bottom of the bag. Fill the bag about half way, shaking the bucket to settle the food. Add another oxygen absorber, and then fill the bucket, leaving about an inch of space on top. Place another oxygen absorber on top.

Pull the bag up as high as you can, settling the food into the bucket. Use a hot iron to seal the Mylar bag. Place a board on the edge of the bucket, lay the bag top straight and start sealing the bag from left to right, making sure to squeeze out excess air before finishing the seal. Fold the bag down, and place the gasket lid on the bucket.

Using Oxygen Absorbers

Oxygen absorbers begin absorbing oxygen the moment they are exposed to air, so don't open your package until you are ready to use them. Remove only the number you need, and immediately place the remaining absorbers in a glass jar with a tight lid.

Rotation

The "Store What You Eat and Eat What You Store" family pantry is a living, breathing organism. It is designed to use

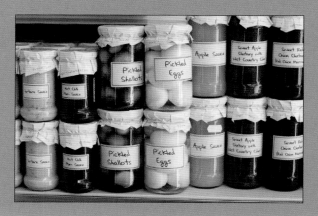

every day, not just in an emergency. Because, for the most part, you are stockpiling foods that are a standard part of your family's diet, you should have an easy time keeping foods fresh and used before their expiration dates.

Always remember FIFO—first in, first out. Develop a system. You can keep older items front and center on your shelf, and fill your shelves from the rear when you add new foods. Or you can store from left to right, always using from the left and adding on the right. Food rotation shelving helps you create an almost foolproof system for your canned goods, feeding them to you in the order you fed them into the shelf.

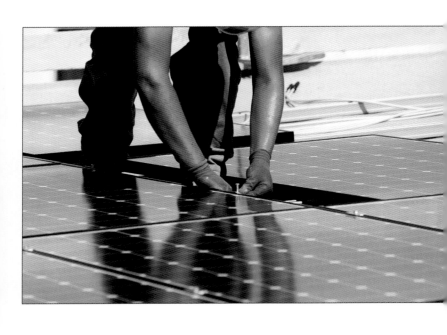

Step 7

Have Access to Alternative Energy Sources

ONE OF THE MOST COMMON FAMILY EMERGEN-cies is the loss of power. How will you heat your home, preserve and cook your food, or provide light without electricity?

Can you name the sources of energy in your house? If you can only name one, you might not be ready in case of an emergency. At our house, we have oil, electricity, propane, and wood. If the power goes out, the oil is pretty much useless because our furnace relies on an electrical blower. So that puts us down to two sources. The propane runs our cooking and our generator, so we could definitely get by for a few days on that. But if problems go on too long, we might be down to wood. That's okay—we can still boil water, cook our food, and stay warm. We have a small woodlot of our own, so we have a reliable supply of wood.

We don't do too much with solar, but it's nice to know the sun is there. We do keep a solar shower out back, and we have a solar oven for drying fruits and vegetables. Oh, and we couldn't

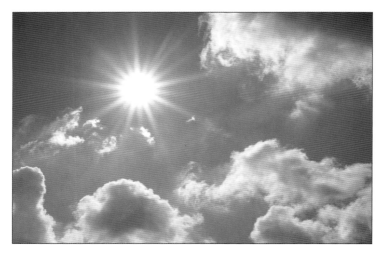

live without our little eighteen-watt solar battery charger for keeping phones and tablets going. Okay, I will add solar power to our list of resources!

Whether you would like to make a short-term emergency cooking plan or figure out long-term alternatives, you should understand all your options.

Fuel Sources

Butane Canister

This fuel is most commonly used in lighters, but can be purchased canned for camping or emergency cooking and heating. Typically reserved for camping and backpacking, this fuel is used with a stove designed specifically for burning butane.

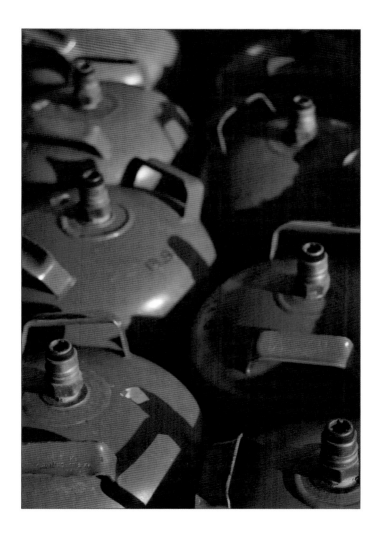

Outside of camping stores, canisters can be hard to find. For short-term emergencies, a butane stove and several canisters can be kept in your storage pantry.

Canned Heat Cell Fuel

Like butane, this fuel is designed for short-term cooking use. Small heat cell fuel cans, such as Sterno, are used with stoves designed especially for use with them. This is a lightweight, easy to store, single-burner solution for emergencies. The fuel is easy to light, and can be relit again and again. It is very stable, so it does not require special storage considerations, and it has an indefinite shelf life. Each can of fuel provides about five hours of cooking time. This simple fuel source is a sensible option to keep with your three-day food supply.

Propane and Natural Gas

Propane and natural gas are great options as long as you can ensure a steady supply for running your generator or emergency stovetop cooking. Because propane is so readily available for home-grilling use, it is relatively easy to purchase and replenish. It is available in small one-pound canisters for emergency use, or in large tanks like the type typically used in gas grills.

If you wish to buy standard grill tanks, consider whether you want the option to refill them at any propane filling station.

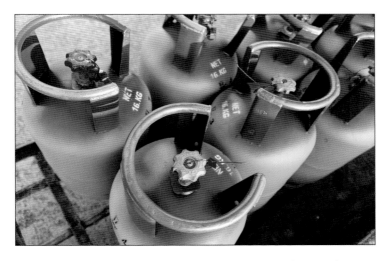

Some propane tank purveyors consider themselves tank-swap suppliers, and have mechanisms that ensure tanks can only be filled by them.

If you already have gas running to your home, you can attach gas appliances and generators to the existing lines.

Usage

Propane tanks are generally measured in pounds. A typical grilling tank is about thirty pounds and holds about seven gallons of fuel.

To calculate how much burn time your tank will provide, first find the empty-tank weight. This number should be engraved on the tank with the letters "TW." Weigh the tank on your bathroom scale and subtract the empty-tank weight from the weight of the canister. The resulting number is the amount of fuel in your tank.

Every pound of propane provides about 21,600 BTUs, but the amount of burn time depends on your stove. Look for the manufacturer's published BTU output to calculate usage for your specific stove or grill. BTU efficiency ranges from 1,000 to 20,000 depending on the type of stove and heat required.

Multiply the pounds of fuel you have in your tank by 21,600. For example, ten pounds of fuel will provide about 216,000 BTUs. Next, check the manufacturer's BTU output for your stove. This number refers to the burn capacity for one hour. If you are using a 10,000 BTU grill, ten pounds of fuel should provide about twenty-one hours of cooking time. Of course, these are just estimates. Actual cooking time depends on a number of factors, but this will help give you a rough idea of your needs.

Storage

Make sure you check that the valve is tight before storing your tank. Because propane is explosive, as well as toxic, store it outside, away from the house. Propane can be stored indefinitely, but there are generally laws regulating how much you can keep on hand, so check your local rulings. It is not safe to bring propane tanks into the house, so use stoves and grills outside only.

Gas Generators

Propane and natural gas generators offer great alternatives to standard gasoline-powered generators. They run cleaner than gasoline, reducing the smell and noise often associated with these generators. There are two kinds of gas-powered generators. Portable-propane generators are attached to your system and used when you need them. These can be used with standard five-gallon propane tanks. Bigger stationary generators are installed units that automatically switch over from electrical to generator when the power goes out.

When choosing a propane or natural gas generator:

* Think about how often you lose power and the degree of inconvenience you are willing to experience.
* Decide on your budget—generators run from hundreds to thousands of dollars. A small portable generator may be fine for infrequent power outages. It works well to power the refrigerator and a few lights. But if you lose your power often or depend on electricity for heating, cooling, and cooking, a permanent standby generator may be worth the expense.
* Identify the electrical items in your home that you want to run on the generator. This will help you decide how large a generator you will need.

- Add up the wattage needed to run the appliances you've chosen, and make sure to include the startup surge required to start the appliance. Plan to run the generator at no more than 50-75 percent of its capacity.
- Consider your options. Portable generators have features that may be worth the added cost, like electric ignition, portability kits, and safety features like high-temperature or low-oil automatic shutdown.

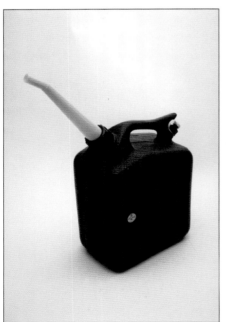

Gasoline

Gasoline is useful for running generators, and a handy supply of it is always welcome for running chainsaws, tractors, and transportation.

Usage

Gasoline comes with a few special problems. First, the shelf life of gasoline is only about six months. If you plan to store it for longer periods, plan on rotating it regularly. A stabilizing agent may be added to extend its life to up to a year, and is a good idea if you will be storing your gasoline in especially warm conditions.

Gasoline requires careful storage. Gasoline should be stored only in approved and specially marked containers, away from the house. Choose a location that is not too warm or near electrical lines or appliances that could ignite it. Do not store gasoline in the basement or utility room.

One gallon of gasoline will provide about 125,000 BTUs. At today's prices, gasoline will run a generator for about twenty-four hours for about half the cost of propane.

Gasoline Generators

Portable generators that run on gasoline are known as inverter generators. Gasoline is used to create DC electricity. Inside the generator is an inverter that converts the DC electricity into AC current, the type of power needed to run household electrical items. Gasoline generators can easily be turned on and off as needed, which makes them handy for intermittent use.

To use your portable gasoline generator:

- Place it on a dry, level surface outdoors. Never use it inside your home, or even your garage. Carbon monoxide fumes released by the generator are deadly.
- Always turn off your generator before refilling it.
- Test your generator regularly by turning it on and running it briefly. Once a month is a good idea. Check batteries and rotate stored gasoline.

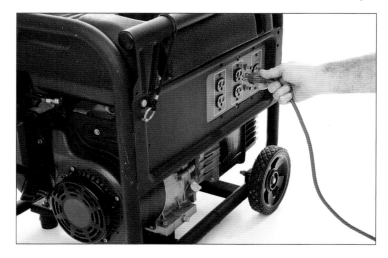

- Invest in a high quality, heavy-duty extension cord for connecting appliances to your portable generator.

Wood and Charcoal

If firewood is readily available, it makes a good source for heat and cooking. Dry hardwood is the best choice; soft woods such as pine and poplar tend to burn too quickly. A wood fire requires about forty-five minutes for coals to reach the proper temperature for cooking. Wood coals tend to be inconsistent in size and do not last as long as charcoal briquettes, so you have to tend the fire more carefully when doing anything but the most basic simmering.

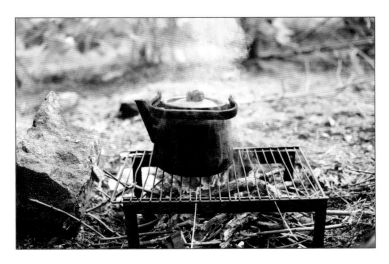

I have found that charcoal briquettes are much easier to use for controlling and maintaining heat. Good charcoal briquettes are a more consistent size than campfire coals, and they burn longer and more evenly. They are easier to move around too, allowing you to adjust your heat quickly and easily.

Usage

Wood and charcoal are not space-saving fuels. To cook for your family for an entire month, you may need 100-200 pounds to provide the needed heat for cooking three meals a day.

Dry wood has about 7,000 BTUs per pound. The drier your wood is and the lower its resin content, the more efficient it will be in producing heat. A good, well-seasoned oak will provide about 24,000,000 BTUs per cord, compared to only 16,000,000 BTUs if you used it green. Compare that to dry white pine, which only provides about 14,000,000 BTUs. Plan on 100–300 pounds of wood to cook for one entire month. Wood usually requires a supply of kindling to get the fire started, so make sure to keep a supply of small combustible pieces readily available.

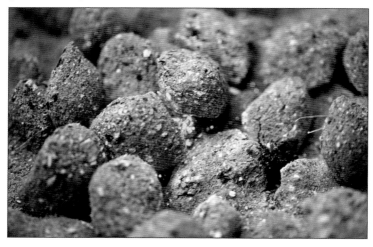

Charcoal provides about 9,000 BTUs per pound. To rely on charcoal for all your cooking for an entire month, you can expect to use about 120–150 pounds. Use a charcoal chimney and paper to start and prepare your charcoals for cooking.

Storage

Cut and split hardwood into 12–18" lengths. Stack wood in a location with plenty of wind and sun so that it has the chance to become dry and well-seasoned. The length of time it takes to season wood depends on weather conditions and seasonality, as well as the wood variety. Winter-cut wood has less sap, so it seasons more easily than summer-cut wood. In general, freshly cut wood should be dried for four to six months

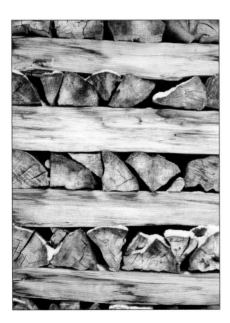

before use. Keep stacked and seasoned wood lightly covered so that the outside surface stays dry. If wood has to remain uncovered, keep bark side up and cut side down, if possible. The drier the wood, the higher its usable energy for burning.

Keep charcoal briquettes in a dry, resealable container to keep them from getting damp and absorbing too much moisture.

Building an Outdoor Fire Pit

To build a fire pit for cooking or staying warm, choose a location with plenty of open space around it. Avoid overhanging branches and roofs that could catch fire, as well as wooden surfaces that might be damaged by falling coals. Dig a shallow hole that is about three feet wide and one foot deep. Line the hole with large flat rocks. Cold earth tends to suck the heat out of a fire, and the rocks will make the pit easier to preheat. Make sure the surface is level—uneven surfaces not only lead to uneven cooking, but with all that hot coal and simmering food, they can be dangerous.

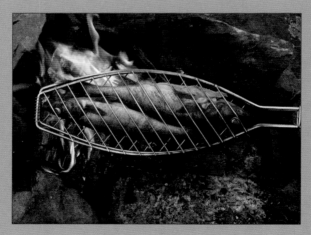

Even a small breeze can play havoc with your cooking temperatures, so carry some kind of shield in your gear to keep out the wind. Any kind of makeshift breeze block will help you

keep your fire burning nicely and prevent ashes from blowing into your food when you lift the lid.

Build your fire of wood or charcoal on top of the rock surface. If cooking with a Dutch oven, place it right in the coals.
Or find a grate to fit over the hole to use for grilling and simmering. Keep a fireplace shovel handy for moving embers and
cleaning out ashes. And don't forget the marshmallows!

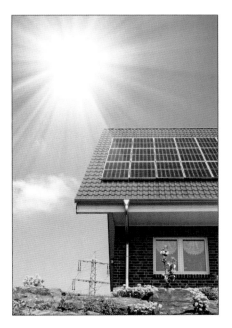

Solar Power

You don't need fancy,
installed solar panels
to take advantage of
the sun. Water can be
heated in a glass jar set
in the sun, and a sim-
ple solar shower can
heat enough water for
a couple of outdoor
showers. A wide array
of recipes can be made
using a solar oven, and
strips of meat, fruits,
and vegetables can be
dried in the sun for
storage. Solar garden

lights take advantage of the daytime sun to provide nighttime lighting for paths and roadways.

Usage

If you are interested in generating solar power to provide all your electrical needs, shop for a photovoltaic panel system. These systems convert the light of the sun to electricity, storing it in batteries for later use. The efficiency of these systems depends upon the amount of sunlight available in your area, so use a map of the United States that outlines sun patterns for different parts of the country.

Before shopping for a solar power system for your home, assess your current usage. Find every way you can to conserve electricity. Change all light bulbs to high-efficiency bulbs. Make sure your water heater is well-insulated and your appliances all meet EnergyStar standards. Next, look at your electric bill to determine how much electricity you use every month, and try to match a system to your usage.

An off-the-grid system can be purchased for a wide range of applications. For a few hundred dollars, a simple eighty-five-watt system can help you keep batteries charged for flashlights, cell phones and other basic needs. Or you can invest tens of thousands of dollars for an 1,800 watt system. Solar power is very appealing for its low impact on the earth, but systems are still very costly and require a fair amount of space to produce adequate power.

Wind Power

To determine whether wind power is practical in your area, consult a United States wind map. Wind maps show whether a turbine would be practical for your location.

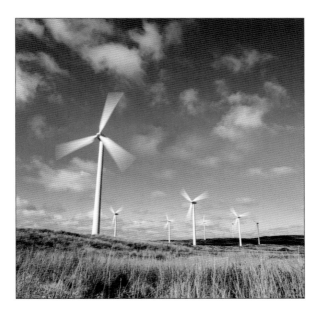

Stand-alone wind turbines are really only practical in rural settings. You need at least an acre of space to get adequate sweep, along with sufficient height (often over sixty feet), to give your turbine the opportunity to produce efficiently.

One wind-powered system that is currently being built for home use combines solar photovoltaic panels with a wind turbine. Because you need steady wind to keep a wind turbine running, it may not be practical for reliable production of power. But here in the United States, where wind speeds may be low in the summer with bright sun, and high in the winter with less sunlight, a system combining the two can keep producing energy all year. To use a system like this, your area requires an average wind speed of about nine miles per hour.

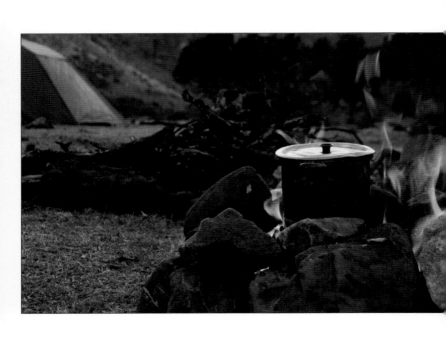

Step 8

Learn to Cook Off the Grid

IF YOU PLAN TO COOK USING AN OUTDOOR propane grill or gas stove, cooking will not be much different than it is inside the house on your kitchen stove. But to get the most out of cooking with alternative forms of fuel, there are a couple of methods that I find particularly useful.

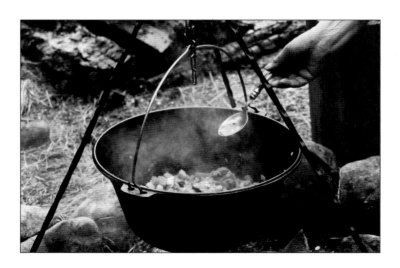

Cooking in a Thermos

This is the simplest possible method of cooking off the grid. With a good quality wide mouth thermos and some boiling water, you can have a hot breakfast waiting for you in the morning.

To make thermos oatmeal, put on a pot of water to boil. Fill the thermos with the hot water and close the lid. Set it aside to warm up.

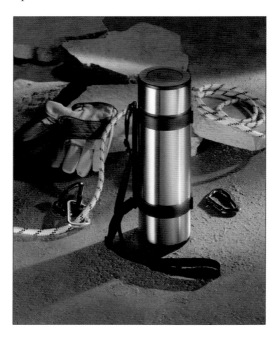

Boil another batch of water. When it is ready, open the thermos and pour out the water. Put one cup of steel-cut oatmeal in the thermos and add about 3.5 cups of boiling water. Close the lid and shake the thermos. Wrap it in a blanket or towel if you like, to help keep it hot. Set it aside. The oatmeal will be ready to eat in less than an hour, but will stay warm all night and be ready to eat in the morning.

This method will work for grains and lentils too. Experiment with a combination of rice, beans, or dried vegetables for a nutritious, hot dinner.

Cooking with a Solar Oven

This is the gentlest and most environmentally friendly method of cooking, nothing but the sun is needed to produce great meals. The solar oven comes in a number of varieties, but it is essentially nothing more than a box that concentrates and traps the heat of the sun. The food inside is gently cooked at a temperature of around 325°F or higher, depending on the intensity of the sun. To cook your food, all you do is place it inside the oven, point it at the sun and wait. Think of it as a natural crock pot.

The solar oven works very well when the sun is in full force, so it is designed for use during the day. The only tending needed is to check and adjust its position every couple of hours to make sure that it is getting the full force of the sun. Because your food won't burn, there is no need to stir or fuss with it during its cooking time. Because no smoke is produced and the gentle heat never reaches dangerous temperatures, the solar oven can be left unattended.

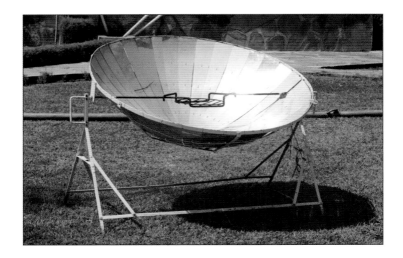

Bright sun is the only requirement for cooking. But even on the sunniest day, cooking times will be affected by factors such as outside temperatures, wind, and elevation, so it may require a bit of experimentation to learn the time needed to cook your food. Smaller batches work best, small cuts of meat rather than large roasts, sliced potatoes instead of whole ones. A small pot of rice will cook in approximately four hours, a simple chili or stew in four or five hours, a small roast in about six hours. The solar oven will bake basic breads or cookies, but they will not brown like a conventional oven.

Great Campfire Coffee

What to do without that electric drip pot? Try this recipe for Egg Coffee!

Fill a pot with ten cups of water and bring it to a boil. In a bowl, combine coffee grounds, egg, and one-fourth cup of water. Stir the egg and coffee mixture into the boiling water and continue to boil for two to three minutes. Before serving, remove from heat and add one cup of cold water. This settles the coffee grounds to the bottom of the pot. Pour a cup, using a strainer if you prefer your coffee without any floating debris.

Why eggs, you ask? I am not sure, although I do know the egg adds body to the coffee and helps to remove any bitterness, leaving you with a smooth, mild cup.

Using a Dutch Oven

When it comes to campfire cooking, there is nothing that compares with the Dutch oven. The Dutch oven is a fryer-broiler-stewer-roaster-steamer-baking oven all-in-one. It is designed to keep moisture in and retain and circulate heat directly around your food. Dutch ovens are designed for outdoor use with wood or charcoal briquettes.

Off-the-grid cooking often means outdoor cooking—and that brings with it a number of factors that have to be considered. Wind, air temperature, humidity, location, and your cooking surface all play a part in how you will generate and maintain your heat. A little wind can gobble up your coals

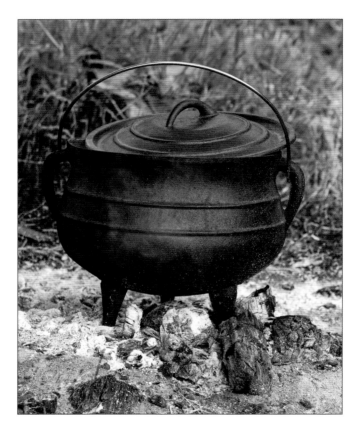

faster than you had planned, high humidity can slow them down, and a shady location or cold ground surface can lower your temperature by twenty-five degrees or more.

Calculating Heat

The Dutch oven is such a versatile cooking unit, it makes sense that there a number of ways to heat and cook with it. Learn to calculate your coal needs based on a few basic rules.

A single charcoal briquette generates around 15°F. That means to maintain a temperature of about 350°F, you would use approximately twenty-four coals. This is handy to know, but not entirely reliable because it doesn't factor in oven size or other conditions. It is just a good starting point. It is always best to be a little conservative when starting out. An overly hot oven can burn your food. It is always easier to build the heat than it is to cool down a hot Dutch oven.

Laying coals for different types of cooking is a matter of ratios. If you are reading a Dutch oven recipe, you may see two numbers. The first number always refers to the coals you will put on top of your oven. The second number is the number of coals you will put on the bottom. For example, 4:1 means four times as many coals on the top of the oven as on the bottom. One the other hand, 1:4 means that there would be four times as many coals on the bottom as on the top. Baking requires a different ratio than roasting, and simmering requires a different ratio than frying. To get the most out of a Dutch oven, learn the basics of regulating temperature.

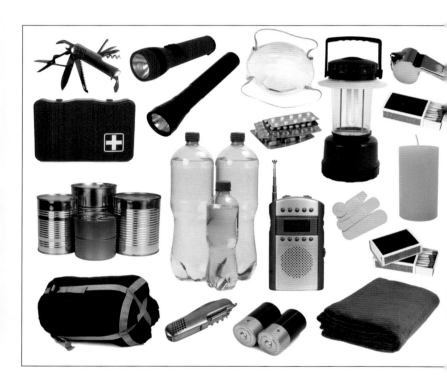

Step 9

Develop Self-Sufficiency

PEOPLE WHO LIVE A MODERN LIFESTYLE MUST depend on someone else for almost everything. Whether it is having the doctor fix every little ache, a foreign factory making your clothes, or Middle Eastern oilfields providing your heat, it may seem almost impossible to develop a self-sustaining lifestyle.

But self-sufficiency is not an all-or-nothing proposition. It does not mean that you have to go it alone. As a matter of fact, in this day and age, it would be extremely unlikely that you would suddenly find yourself in remote backwoods with no one to depend upon but yourself.

There is a lot of value in knowing how to provide and preserve food, keep everyone safely sheltered, and rely on your own resources to take care of your family. So strive to be a little more self-sufficient today than you were yesterday. If you are entirely dependent on outside resources, aim for 10 percent self-sufficiency. If that works out, look for ways to be 20 percent self-sufficient. Decide how you want to spend your time and resources. Some people are content to stockpile food. Others want to grow and preserve their own. Still others find it fulfilling to seek out

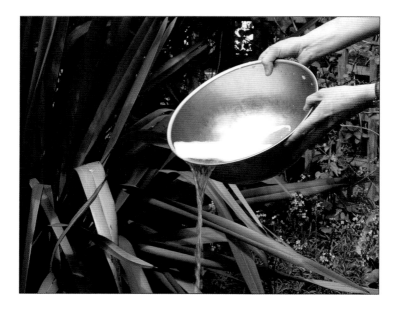

and barter for local goods, foods, and services. All of these things help loosen the stranglehold the world has on your life.

Keep Germs at Bay

The most important rule of the prepper—keep yourself healthy. That means making sure you do not unnecessarily expose yourself to anything that could make you sick. Make sure you have a good plan for handling basic sanitation needs in the event of loss of power or water supplies, and know how to keep food and water supplies safe.

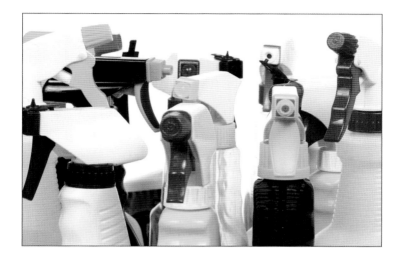

The very best way to reduce or prevent the spread of illness is to keep your hands clean. Germs accumulate on your hands as you go throughout your day, and even the most innocent of objects may carry your next cold.

How to Wash Your Hands

Always wash your hands BEFORE preparing or eating food, or anytime you have to care for a sick or injured person.

Always wash your hands AFTER handling raw meat, using the bathroom or changing a diaper, blowing your nose, treating a sick or injured person, or anytime your hands get dirty or you handle contaminated materials.

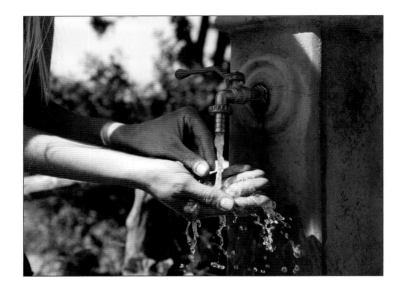

To wash your hands:
- Wet hands with warm water and add soap.
- Rub your hands together for about twenty seconds, making sure to scrub all surfaces, including the back of the hand, between fingers, wrists, and under nails. (This takes about as long as it takes to sing Happy Birthday twice.)
- Rinse hands thoroughly with warm running water.
- If you are in a public location, dry your hands with a paper towel. Use that towel to turn off the water and open the door before discarding.

- If water is not available, use a hand sanitizer that contains at least 60 percent alcohol. Your hands may not actually be clean, but they should be more or less sterile.

Baking Soda!

Baking soda is good for more than baking. It is great for deodorizing almost anything, works as an acid neutralizer, and can even stop an itch.

- Mix it in your bath water for a deodorizing cleanse.
- Make a paste with it for brushing your teeth and freshening your breath.
- Stir a little soda into water to make a soothing drink to counteract an upset stomach.

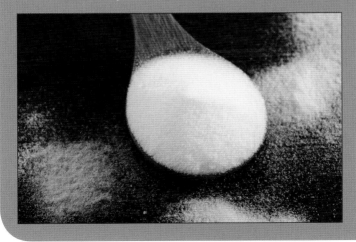

- Use a dash of baking soda under the arms as a replacement for deodorant.
- Apply a paste of baking soda and water to stings and bites to reduce itching.
- Add baking soda to laundry to eliminate smells and loosen stains.
- A little baking soda instead of powder in the diaper can help neutralize ammonia.

Get Immunized!

Vaccines have been the subject of controversy in the news, particularly as to how they impact childhood development. But the fact is that vaccines are the best defense we have against some of the most common serious and even deadly contagious diseases. Childhood vaccines are generally mandated by law in order for children to attend school, but if you have special concerns, discuss them with your doctor.

Adults should also discuss with their physicians what vaccines they need to maintain. For example, an up-to-date tetanus vaccine can remove worry about puncture wounds or other dirty skin wounds. The good news is that a booster shot lasts ten years, so updating it is not a real hardship. Flu shots may be appropriate for anyone who cannot afford an extended illness or is caring for children or seniors. Seniors may want to protect themselves from shingles, pneumonia, or whooping cough, which can take a greater toll on an older body.

Build a First Aid Kit

Make up a complete first aid kit of your own, containing enough of the basics to get you through just about anything. Tailor it for any special needs of your family. Even more importantly, KNOW HOW TO USE IT. Take a class in first aid and CPR from your college's continuing education department or your local hospital.

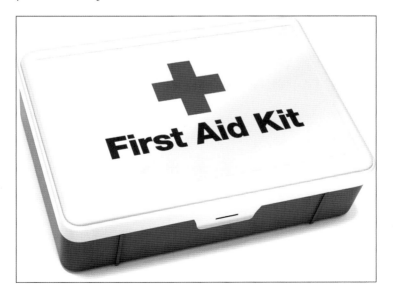

A good kit includes:

- Burn ointment
- Triple antibiotic cream
- Hydrogen peroxide
- Benzalkonium chloride
- Adhesive bandages
- Small splints
- Gauze
- First aid tape
- Small scissors
- Tweezers
- Sterile cotton balls and swabs
- Matches
- Thermometer
- Cold medicine
- Antacids
- Antibiotics
- Antidiarrheal medicine
- Syrup of ipecac
- Antihistamines
- Laxatives
- Multi-vitamins
- Petroleum jelly
- Prescription medicines
- Heavy string
- Sunscreen
- Aloe cream

Take Vitamins

The best way to be healthy is to stay healthy. Store multi-vitamins for everyone in your household, and make sure that you have vitamin C on hand as well. Keeping your immune system strong will help you avoid many of the most common illnesses.

Stock Prescriptions

Make sure you have an extra one- to three-month supply of any necessary prescription drugs that the family takes. Get a few months extra and keep it in your surplus personal stock, making sure to rotate it to keep it fresh.

Some people try to stockpile antibiotics. Be cautious about administering antibiotics. Although they are potential lifesavers, misuse or overuse can get you into trouble. If you think you need an antibiotic, see a doctor.

Have an Extra Set of Eyeglasses

Make sure you have an extra set of eyeglasses for anyone in the family who uses them. Anytime you get new glasses, save previous eyeglasses in your first aid kit in case of emergencies or breakage, or take advantage of the two-for-one deals that many eyeglass companies offer.

Prepare for Dental Emergencies

The best defense against dental emergencies is a good offense. Make sure that your family keeps up a good regimen of brushing and flossing to keep teeth and gums in prime condition. Avoid excessive amounts of highly-acidic foods that can weaken tooth enamel. If you do eat high-acid foods, don't run straight to the bathroom to brush your teeth. Acid actually softens enamel, so immediate brushing may do more harm than good. Wait at least an hour before you brush.

Let your kids chew sugar-free gum with xylitol. It helps to reduce acid and increase saliva flow. Saliva actually helps prevent enamel erosion by strengthening teeth with key minerals.

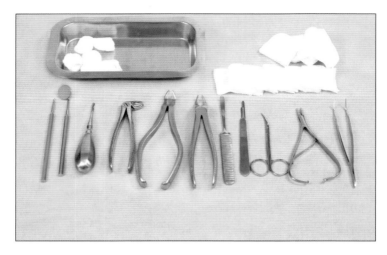

Keep fluoride toothpaste in your pantry, along with a supply of extra toothbrushes. Toothbrushes should actually be replaced every three months or so, more often if you have gum disease.

Plan for dental emergencies by having a few key items in your healthcare cupboard. These items might include:

- Cotton rolls
- Dental mirror
- Sterile gauze pads
- Temporary filling material
- Crown cement
- Oral anesthetic for treating gum or tooth pain
- Floss, mouthwash, and dental picks

Control Aches and Pains

Know how to handle the everyday aches and pains of work and exercise. Paying attention to minor aches and strains will help you to avoid overusing a joint that is sending out warning signals!

How do you know whether to use heat or cold on your aching joints?

Use ice packs immediately after an acute injury or to treat joints immediately after a workout. Ice helps to reduce swelling and limit internal bleeding. Ice an injured joint for ten minutes at a time. Let the skin return to a normal temperature, and then repeat the icing, up to three times. Do this for one to three days after an injury.

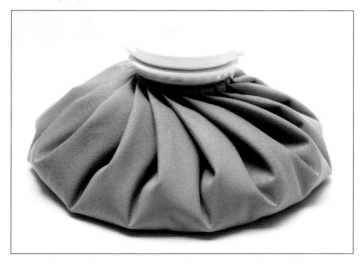

Heat therapy is used for chronic aching joints and stiffness, and is useful for arthritic conditions. Heat can be used before exercise to help loosen stiff joints and is great for relaxing tight muscles and treating spasms. Use warm, damp towels or warm therapy packs, and leave on the joint for fifteen to twenty minutes. Moist heat combined with eucalyptus ointment makes an especially comforting treatment. Just rub ointment onto the joint, wrap the area in plastic wrap, and leave in place for about twenty minutes. Note: never use heat on an inflamed or swollen joint, or immediately after exercise.

Your aches-and-pains kit should include:

- Ibuprofen
- Hot water bottle
- Hot and cold therapy packs
- Freezer gel packs
- Moleskin pads
- Elastic bandages
- Rubbing alcohol
- Eucalyptus ointment
- Epsom salt
- Elastic bandages

Basic First Aid

Assist Choking Victims

Choking is caused when the airway is partially or completely blocked by a piece of food or another object. When the airway is partially blocked, a person may be able to cough out the offending object. Stay with them until the choking is resolved.

But when the airway is completely blocked, the person will not be able to speak, cough, or breathe. Learn the Heimlich maneuver to assist someone in this condition.

1 Stand behind the choking person, and wrap your arms around his waist.

2 Make a fist and place the thumb side of your fist against his upper abdomen, below the ribcage and above the navel.

3 Place your other hand over your fist and press into his upper abdomen with a quick, upward thrust.

4 Repeat until the object is dislodged and the person can catch a breath.

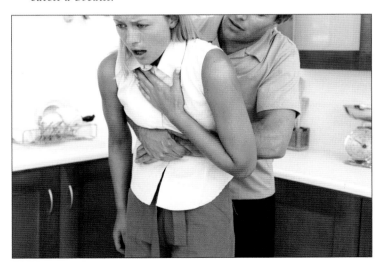

For a young child:

Lay the child on his back and position yourself facing him. Place the middle and index fingers of both hands below the rib cage but above the navel. Gently press into the upper abdomen with a quick, upward thrust. Repeat until the object is dislodged and the child can catch a breath.

For a baby:

Sit the infant or toddler on your lap facing away from you and place the middle and index fingers of both hands below the rib cage but above the navel. Gently press into the upper abdomen with a quick, upward thrust. Repeat until the object is dislodged and the child can catch a breath.

If you are alone and choking:

If you can't speak or breathe, there may not be time to seek assistance from someone else. Make a fist and place it against your upper abdomen, just below the ribcage. Grasp your fist with your other hand and press into your upper abdomen with a quick, upward thrust. If you cannot gain enough traction, press your abdomen against the back of a chair or the side of a table to produce an upper thrust. Repeat until the object is dislodged and you can catch a breath.

CPR

If at all possible, take a CPR training course. The American Heart Association, the American Red Cross, and many hospitals and fire departments offer courses and can provide more thorough instructions.

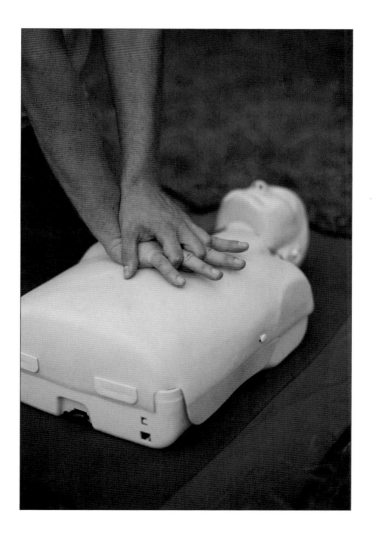

If you do run into a situation where immediate assistance is required, do the following:

- Call 911 immediately if a person is clearly in distress or unresponsive.
- If the person is not breathing normally, cannot cough, or is not moving, start chest compressions by pushing down in the center of the chest. Press hard and fast—your rate should be at least 100 pumps per minute, or almost twice per second. Press about two inches down and repeat thirty times.
- Tilt the person's head back and lift the chin. Pinch the nose and cover the mouth with yours. Blow in two breaths of about one second each. You should be able to see the chest rise.
- Repeat the pattern of thirty pumps and two breaths until help arrives. If the person starts to vomit, turn the head to the side and try to clear the mouth.

Stop the Bleeding

If bleeding occurs due to a cut or other traumatic injury, there is only one step. Stop the bleeding. Put direct pressure on the wound immediately. If you can get some clean gauze or a towel, place that over the wound and hold it down tightly. If the gauze bleeds through, just add more on top. Don't peel it away, as that will cause the bleeding to begin again. Once the bleeding is under control, clean and bandage the wound. If bleeding begins again, reapply pressure until it is under control again. If bleeding is severe, watch for signs of shock. Lay the

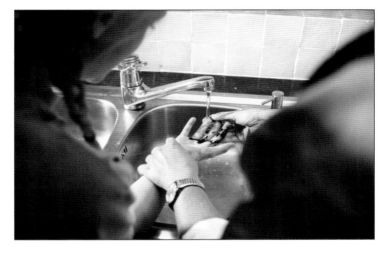

person flat, cover with a blanket, and keep the injured area above heart level if possible.

Treat Cuts

When it comes to minor cuts and scrapes, keep it simple. Even small cuts can bleed heavily, so if there is significant bleeding, first apply pressure to reduce the flow. Wash the wound with soap and water and apply an elastic bandage, being careful that it is not tight enough to cut off circulation. Before bedtime, change the bandage, making it a little looser than the daytime bandage. Do this twice a day until the wound has stabilized and the bandage can be removed. The most important thing is to keep the wound dry; do not use first aid ointment, and change the bandage if the wound area gets wet.

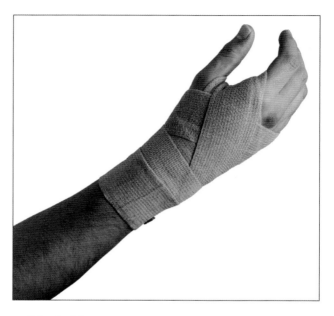

Stop a Bloody Nose

Whether from a good whack in the nose or simply dry nasal passages—when a nose decides to bleed, it may take a little time and patience to get it under control. Follow these steps:

- Have the person lean forward so that any dripping blood leaves the body, rather than going down the throat.
- Find the area just below the bridge and pinch the nose together firmly. Hold it for a full five minutes; it may take that much time for the blood to clot. If you can, add a cold compress just above the bridge to help constrict the blood vessels.

- If the nose is still bleeding after five minutes, pinch and hold again. This time wait ten minutes before releasing. If you still cannot get the bleeding under control, see a doctor.

   If a head injury occurred but there is no sign of facial injury, a bloody nose may be a sign of a more serious situation. Contact a physician immediately.

Treat Burns

Burns are very common around the home, and quick action really helps to lessen the pain! For minor burns, the first thing to do is get the affected area under cold running water. It doesn't have to be icy to reduce the pain. If you don't have running water, use a cold compress. Once the pain subsides, cover the burn with a sterile bandage. Give acetaminophen or ibuprofen for pain. Do not break a blister or use ointment on the burn.

   If a burn is severe, cool and cover the burn, and then watch for signs of shock. Lay the person flat and cover with a blanket. Elevate the burn above the heart.

Remove Ticks

Ticks are more than a nuisance; they can carry Lyme disease. If you get a tick bite, you need to remove it as soon as you can. Don't try to smother or get the tick to back out using petroleum jelly or rubbing alcohol. This may actually cause the tick to release toxins into your system.

   Avoid the temptation to grab the tick with your fingers and yank. Instead, take the time to get a good pair of tweezers. Carefully grab the tick as close to your skin as possible. Don't

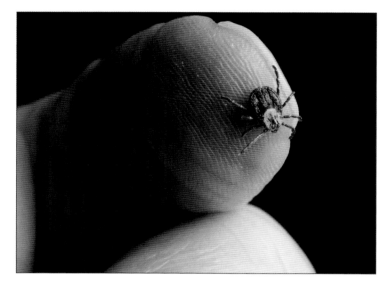

twist it, just pull gently until it detaches. Look at the tick to make sure you got the whole thing. If not, try to remove the head from the skin with your tweezers. Clean the wound with rubbing alcohol, and then wash your hands thoroughly with soap and water.

If a rash develops around the bite site, or fever or flu-like symptoms occur within weeks of the bite, see a doctor to be checked for Lyme disease.

Dealing with Bee Stings

People often get multiple bee stings, because bees just seem to know when to call in the cavalry! So if you get a bee sting, the first thing to do is get out of there! Bees will even give chase, so don't stop until you know you are out of their path. Then check the sting. If the stinger is still there, remove it by pulling it out quickly. Place ice on the sting immediately. Pain, itching, and swelling are common. A paste of baking soda and water applied to the sting may bring some relief.

Watch for signs of a more serious reaction called anaphy-laxis. If the person has been stung more than ten times or if there is shortness of breath or tightening of the throat, seek professional help immediately. An antihistamine like Benadryl can help slow the reaction, but it is still best to have the person checked out by a doctor. Ibuprofen or acetaminophen can be given for pain.

Note: if the person has an identified bee allergy and car-ries an EpiPen, help him administer the injection immediately before symptoms appear!

Animal Bites

The best way to handle animal bites is to avoid them. Animals carry a number of diseases; even domestic animals' mouths can transfer harmful bacteria. Do your best to prevent animal bites by wearing long pants and boots in areas of heavy brush. Never approach a wild animal or unfamiliar domestic pet. Make sure tetanus shots are up to date, and get a booster if you are unsure of when your last one was given.

If someone has been bitten by an animal, thorough clean-ing is required. Get bleeding under control first by applying

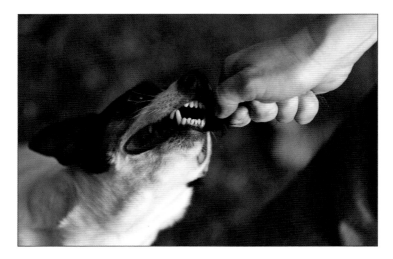

pressure to the wound. If the bite is on the hand, remove any rings or jewelry that could become stuck in the event of swelling. Flush out the wound with soap and water. Apply antibiotic cream and cover with a sterile bandage. Keep the wound clean by changing the bandage twice a day, and reapplying antibiotic cream. Puncture wounds may be harder to clean thoroughly, and need to be watched for signs of infection.

Signs of infection such as heat, redness, and swelling require additional care. If fever or increased pain occurs, antibiotics may be needed. See a doctor if the bite area fails to heal normally.

Remove a Splinter
Splinters of any kind are irritating, and depending on what kind they are, can cause infection if left in the skin. Wash

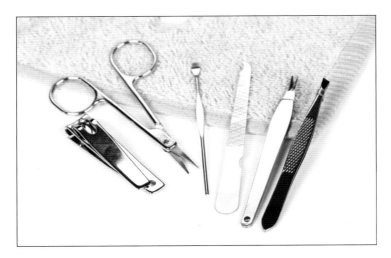

your hands thoroughly before attempting to remove the splinter. Clean a needle and a pair of tweezers with povidone-iodine or isopropyl alcohol. Clean the area around the splinter with soap and water, and wipe it down with the iodine solution.

If the splinter end is protruding, try to gently grasp it with tweezers and pull it out of the skin. A little pushing around the sides and bottom of the splinter may help raise it to the surface.

If the entire splinter is under the skin, open the skin gently using the needle. When you have exposed the splinter, use the tweezers to grasp and remove it. Clean the area again and inspect for signs of any slivers left behind. Wipe down the site with povidone-iodine.

Treat Soft Tissue Injuries

Use the **R-I-C-E** method for dealing with simple soft tissue injuries, like pulls or sprains.

Rest: Stop using the injured area for forty-eight hours.

Ice: Put an ice pack on the injured area for twenty minutes at a time, four to eight times per day.

Compression: Use an elastic bandage to provide compression for an injured ankle, knee, or wrist. This will help to reduce the swelling.

Elevation: Keep the injured area elevated above the level of the heart. Use a pillow to help elevate an injured limb.

Treat the Common Cold

There is nothing common about the common cold. In fact, the common cold isn't just one condition. There are actually hundreds of different viruses that are responsible for the symptoms we associate with a cold.

Colds are just one of those annoyances of life—no matter how hard you try, one is going to catch up with you every now and then. Prevention is all about keeping your hands clean and avoiding direct exposure to coughing or sneezing. Anything that negatively impacts your immune system will make you more susceptible to colds, so eat well, exercise and get enough sleep, avoid smoking and pollutants, and try to keep stress at manageable levels to keep your body's resistance high.

If you do succumb to a cold, expect about seven days of symptoms. There is an old saying that it takes two days to get a cold, three days to have a cold, and two days to get rid of a cold. If you have symptoms for a lot longer than that, or if your symptoms worsen just when they should be getting better, you may be dealing with more than a cold. Antibiotics are of no use in treating colds, but may be indicated if symptoms worsen and indicate the presence of a bacterial infection.

Because there is nothing you can do to get rid of a cold, the goal of treatment is to make you more comfortable. Drink plenty of fluids to loosen phlegm and flush toxins out of your system. Gargle with salt water to ease a sore throat, and use nasal saline drops to relieve stuffiness. Use a humidifier to moisten the air in your home, and try eucalyptus to ease congestion. Oh, and your mom was right, chicken soup helps.

Take pain relievers for head and body aches. If you want to take cold medicine, make sure you match your medicine to the symptoms. If in doubt, ask the pharmacist for a recommendation. Don't accidentally overdose yourself on pain remedies. Many cold medications already contain pain relievers so don't add another round of acetaminophen or ibuprofen to your regimen. An overdose of acetaminophen can damage the liver, causing a life-threatening situation.

Be cautious about giving children cold medication. Many over-the-counter medications are not safe for children under four. Try to keep young children occupied and comfortable, and see a doctor if there is a fever of more than 102°F, you see symptoms of dehydration, ear pain, or thick green mucous discharge.

Counteract Nausea

Nausea is that queasy I–feel–yucky sensation you get in the stomach. Often you feel the need to vomit, and may feel shaky, sweaty, or crampy. Nausea is not an illness in itself. It tends to be a symptom of some other type of condition. Motion sickness, pregnancy, migraines, flu, even bad smells can trigger nausea. Occasionally, nausea also signals a more serious condition like appendicitis, food poisoning, a bad reaction to medication, or even heart attack.

When nausea strikes, rest quietly, but do not lay down flat. Instead, rest in a reclining position. Drink clear fluids and nibble on bland foods like saltine crackers or plain bread. Eat very lightly, with small meals throughout the day. Cold foods also seem to be more agreeable than hot foods, and as you start to feel better you may have a desire for something salty or acidic. Avoid strong cooking smells, fatty foods, and stuffy rooms.

Ginger is considered a good home remedy for nausea. Nibbling on candied ginger or even smelling ginger can be helpful. Some people like peppermint, citrus, or chamomile teas.

Nausea should not last very long. If you continue to experience symptoms of nausea for several days, see a physician. There are medications to help control symptoms, but it is important to understand the underlying cause of extended bouts of nausea.

Stop Diarrhea

A bout of diarrhea may be no more than an annoyance, but if it goes on too long, it can quickly turn serious, particularly for children. The greatest danger with diarrhea is dehydration and loss of electrolytes. The most important thing for someone who is experiencing diarrhea to do is to keep hydrated. Provide clear broth, chamomile tea, water, or electrolyte drinks. Avoid milk, apple juice, alcohol, or caffeine products, which may make symptoms worse. A bout of diarrhea should be considered serious if it goes on longer than twenty-four hours in children and two to three days in adults.

Antidiarrheal medicines are not necessarily the way to go. First, whatever it is that caused the problem is trying to flush itself out of the system, and that's a good thing. Second, antidiarrheal medicines can cause more problems than they fix—turning that steady stream into constipation. If you need immediate relief, know what the various medicines do. Kaopectate absorbs fluid, while Imodium slows the action of the gut. Pepto-bismol seems to work at soothing the gut and may kill some of the bad bacteria. Get advice from your doctor about the best choice for children.

When symptoms start to subside, ease back into solid food slowly. Try starchy, low fiber foods like bananas, rice, applesauce, or white toast. Avoid fatty or high fiber foods. Once the worst has passed, add some live culture yogurt to the diet to help get the good bacteria back into the gut.

Grow a Garden

If you live in the country, chances are you already do some form of gardening. But if you live in the city, or even in the suburbs, you may not feel that you have the space to produce enough fruit and vegetables to be worth your while. The reality is, though, that even a small well-designed garden can produce enough to supplement your family's diet.

You can build a raised-bed garden in as little as four square feet. Square-foot gardening allows you to plant a different crop in each square foot of the garden. Four square feet gives you sixteen different options, and will allow you to grow as much as you might produce in a garden over four times that big. What you put in each square depends on the spacing requirements of the plants you choose. You may put in one tomato in a square foot, or use it to plant nine green bean seeds. If you have more space, you can add additional boxes.

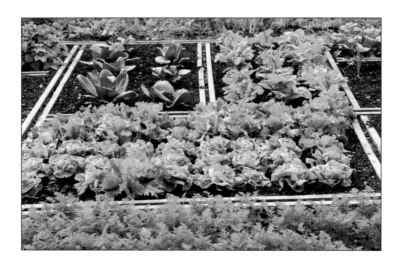

Choose a space for your garden that gets at least six to eight hours of sunshine. Soil quality doesn't matter because you will be building over the location and adding your own blend of soil.

- To create your garden, lay it out in squares that are no larger than four feet. If you are going to have more than one square, make room between them for walking. You will not be stepping into your squares once they are built.

- Construct boxes of 1x6 or 2x6 boards, connected at each corner with deck screws or corner brackets. Try to set the frames as level as possible, using soil to build up low areas. If you are positioning your boxes over grass or a weedy area, cover the ground with landscape paper or plastic to deter weeds.

- Mix a blend of equal parts vermiculite, peat moss, and compost. This blend is very light and will hold moisture very well—especially important in a raised-bed garden that can dry out faster than a conventional one.

- Once your boxes are in place, divide the box into sixteen squares using thin wooden or plastic strips. These grids will help you keep your seeding plan organized. Without it, you will find yourself going outside the lines, planting in rows, or wasting space.

- Choose and plant your vegetable choices. To understand how many seeds or plants to use per square, check the spacing recommendations on the package. Seeds that call for 6" spacing can be planted four per square; those calling for 4" spacing can have nine per square. Plant one or two seeds in each spot, covering lightly with soil.

- Water every day when you first get started. After that, you may only need to water daily when it is very hot. Water early or late, rather than the middle of the day when the sun can evaporate the water quickly.

- Harvest your crops as they come in. If a square gets emptied, replant it with another crop. If there is a threat of frost, it is easy to construct posts to support the addition of a plastic cover over the box. This will turn it into a little hothouse, and help to extend your growing season.

Preserving Your Food

If you grow your own vegetables and fruits, or even if you are just a frequent visitor to the farmer's market, you may want

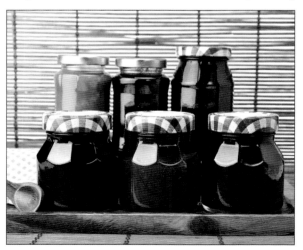

to learn to preserve your own produce. Preserving it yourself allows you to customize salt and sweetening preferences to your family's needs, and lets you put up your favorite jam and pickle recipes. A shelf of home-canned foods is a very rewarding sight, and there is nothing like reaching for your own garden tomatoes on a cold winter's night.

Water Bath Canning

Canning of high-acid produce, such as tomatoes and fruits, requires nothing more than a large water bath canner, along with canning jars with jar lids and screw bands. To can jams, jellies, pickles, fruit, and tomato products, follow these steps:

- Wash jars in hot, soapy water and set aside to drain. Fill the water bath canner with water and set it on the stove to simmer. Place jars on the rack and lower into hot water. The water does not have to boil.

- Place the new jar lids (never reuse jar lids) in a small saucepan, add water, and simmer on the stove. Screw bands should be clean, but do not have to be sterilized.

- Prepare your ingredients and make your recipe, if one is called for.

- When you are ready to fill jars, work with one at a time. Take a hot jar from the pot and pour the water in the jar back into the pot. Using a jar funnel, fill the jar to within ¼"–½" of headspace.

- Using a chopstick or other nonmetallic utensil, stir the ingredients of the jar so that they settle and any air bubbles are released. If you need to add more ingredients or liquid to raise the level after settling, do so now.

- Using a clean cloth, wipe down the rim of the jar so that there is nothing to interfere with the seal. Center a hot jar lid on the top of the jar, and tighten on a screw band by hand. Place the jar back into the water. Repeat until all the jars are filled.

- When the jars are all filled and in the canner, add hot water until the level is about one inch over the top of the jars. Cover, turn up the heat, and bring to a full rolling boil. When the water is boiling, begin counting the processing time. The water should continue to boil during the entire processing period.

- When the processing time is over, turn off the heat and remove the canner lid. Let jars sit inside for about five minutes, and then remove to a towel-covered counter to cool.

- Wait several hours before checking to see whether your jars have sealed properly. To do this, remove the screw band and press down on the center of the lid. It should be slightly concave and should not move when touched. The edge should hold tightly when pressure is applied. If a jar does not seal, just place it in the refrigerator and use within a few days.

- Store sealed and labeled jars in a cool, dark place. Home-canned goods are best used within one year.

- To can low-acid vegetables or meats, a similar procedure is followed, but jars are processed in a pressure cooker to expose them to higher heat that can kill harmful bacterial spores. To can low-acid foods, read the pressure cooker manufacturer's directions, and follow recipe instructions for processing times.

Drying Fruits and Vegetables

Start with fresh, healthy, ripened produce. Remove any produce that is past its prime or shows signs of bruising or other damage.

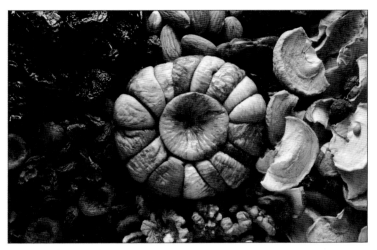

To sun-dry produce:

If your climate provides hot, sunny conditions and relatively low humidity for most of the day, consider sun-drying your produce.

Cut fruit into uniformly sized pieces. Fruit will darken as it dries, so presoak in an ascorbic acid solution before you place on drying racks. To make fruit leather, follow a recipe for a fruit puree, then pour puree onto plastic wrap-lined sheet trays, and dry as you would fruit slices.

You can use a window screen as your drying rack if you like. Place fruit cut-side down and lay out in the sun as early in the day as you can so you can take advantage of the most sun. A porch roof or a truck bed is ideal, and will concentrate the heat to make drying much faster. A solar oven would also produce concentrated heat.

Cover racks with a light mesh fabric. Allow produce to dry on one side all day. At night, cover the screens with a light sheet, or bring inside if you think the evening will be cool or damp. The next day, turn produce over and repeat the process. Sun drying may take up to three days to complete. Dried fruit should be leathery but still flexible.

Most vegetables are best sliced as thin chips. When vegetables are clean and sliced, blanch them lightly in boiling water before beginning the drying process. This helps set the color and preserve many of the vitamins. When vegetables are ready, lay them out and dry as you would fruit.

To oven-dry produce:

In cooler or more humid conditions, oven-drying provides a more reliable method for producing consistently good dried fruits and vegetables.

Turn your oven onto the lowest heat setting, about 200°F. Slice the produce, stemming and removing seeds if necessary. Place on cookie sheets and leave them in the oven all day or overnight. Check them occasionally, rotating the sheets and turning over slices as needed. Larger pieces can take as much as forty-eight hours to reach the perfect dryness, but most will be done within twenty-four hours.

Dehydrators can also be used for drying. Dehydrators require electricity and have relatively low capacity, but are very convenient for processing small batches.

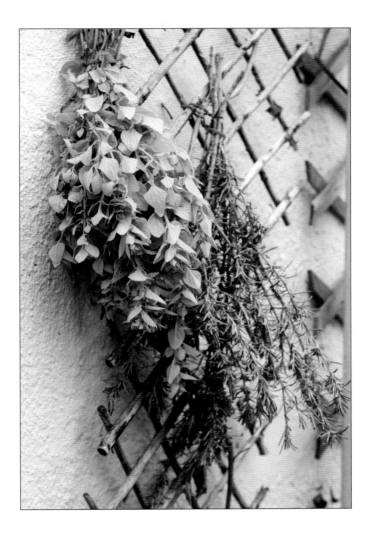

Air-Drying Herbs

Fresh herbs are too delicate for direct sunlight, but can easily be air-dried. Harvest and wash your herbs on the stems. Lay them out to dry on a towel. Then gather them into a bunch and tie the stems together. Hang the bunch upside down in a warm, dry place with good air circulation. Drying takes five or more days, depending on humidity and temperature conditions. Store dried herbs in airtight containers.

Making Jerky

Start with two pounds of a lean cut of meat, like sirloin or a round steak. (It will be easier to work with if you freeze it slightly.) Trim all visible fat; lean jerky will keep better than fatty strips. Slice into very thin strips. Cut against the grain for a more tender jerky, with the grain for a chewier style.

If you want to flavor your meat, marinate it using a recipe created for jerky. I like soy sauce with garlic, salt, and just a dash of Tabasco, but this step is optional and I often skip it.

A good rub is important though. My rub consists of two teaspoons of kosher salt, one teaspoon of black pepper, one teaspoon of garlic powder, and one tablespoon of brown sugar. Add some cayenne if you want a little kick. Coat your meat with this rub and refrigerate for twelve to twenty-four hours.

Another way to prepare your jerky is to combine your rub spices into your marinade. Marinate overnight and then dry your jerky. Check out jerky recipes and try one that sounds good to you.

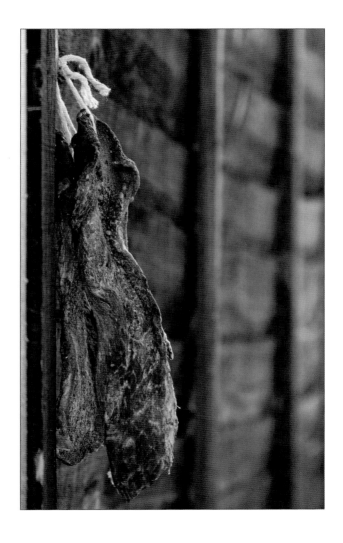

Place your prepared meat on a broiler pan or a wire rack over a sheet tray, and place inside an oven set at about 200°F (a little lower if your oven goes below 200°F). Watch it carefully. If the heat is too low, it won't kill the bacteria. If it is too high, it will cook the meat rather than drying it out. If you have a dehydrator, follow the manufacturer's instructions.

Bake for four to six hours, or until jerky is dry to the touch and a nice, dark brown inside. Cool at room temperature, and store in sealable plastic bags.

Keeping Chickens

If you want to have a steady supply of eggs, and are not squeamish about processing your own meat, you may find that raising chickens is a rewarding addition to your sustainable lifestyle.

Backyard eggs contain one-third of the cholesterol of store-bought eggs and more vitamin A, vitamin E, beta carotene, and Omega-3. Home-grown eggs are much more flavorful and richly colored than anything you will find in the grocery store. A family of four needs only a small flock to provide all the eggs it can use.

You can start your own chicken flock by buying chicks at the local feed store or farm supplier.

The first sixty days are crucial. Young chicks need to be kept warm and given clean bedding and a safe place to get some fresh air.

After sixty days, or when your chicks are feathered out, it is time to move them into a coop. Your chicken coop should

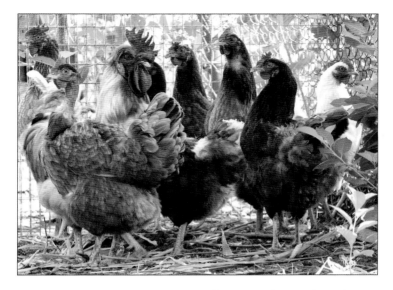

be designed to protect chickens from weather and predators. There should be perches comfortable for perching and roosting. You should plan on about two to three square feet of indoor space for each chicken and four to five feet of outdoor run space per chicken.

Before embarking on a chicken project, get to know others in the area that raise chickens, and read up on all the ins and outs of being a chicken farmer. You may find that raising chickens may lead to goats and rabbits and your own honey bees. Or you may discover that raising chickens is not for you, but meet others with whom you can barter for fresh eggs and organic meat.

Bartering

It can be very liberating to know that you can get what you want without using money. Bartering is as simple as trading what you want for what someone else needs. Start by figuring out what you have that may be of value to someone else. Maybe you grow terrific tomatoes but are wishing you had fresh eggs. If you can find a chicken farmer who doesn't spend a lot of time in his garden, you may have a deal. He may even be willing to trade you some of that wonderful manure he is producing in exchange for a portion of next year's crop.

Perhaps you are a great bookkeeper or know how to design and maintain websites. And maybe you like the food at a particular restaurant. A deal may be mutually beneficial.

Maybe you make great pies and your friend makes wonderful baked beans. Perhaps all the guys are handy, and can start a home repair team to help each other with projects. Once you start thinking in this way, the possibilities are endless.

Once you find a like-minded person who is willing to trade goods or services, hammer out the details. If you are just swapping those tomatoes for eggs, a handshake may suffice. But for many trades, it is best to put the details in writing, particularly if you are trading for services. Designate what you will do and what you will receive. Set how much time will be allocated to it and name a deadline to complete services.

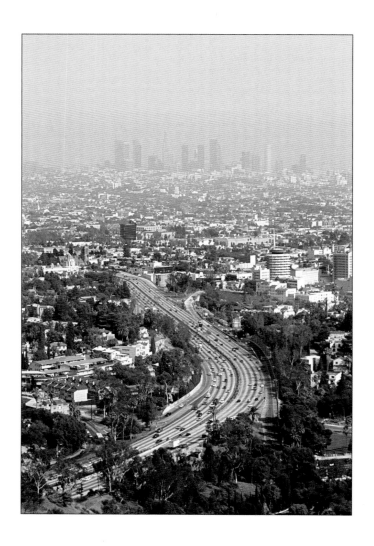

Step 10

Know When to Go— The Art of Evacuation

YOU MAY THINK THAT WITH ALL YOUR preparation, home is the safest place to be. And in most cases you are probably correct. But sometimes the only answer is to get out. When public service announcements require evacuation, don't ignore them. Mandatory evacuations are not issued lightly.

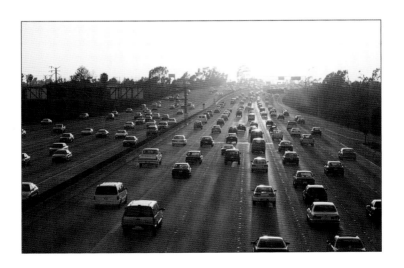

If you have time, turn off appliances and electronics, and shut down utilities if the situation warrants it. Shut windows and doors, grab your go-bags, and lock up when you leave.

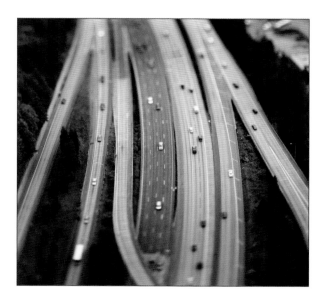

Maintaining Your Vehicle

Your car may be your lifeline if it comes time to outrun a storm or other emergency. Learn to know it as well as you know your home. It provides shelter, transportation, and allows you to reach goods and services you may not have available at home.

Like you, your car thrives on being well cared for. Learn its maintenance needs, and understand the basics of filters, belts, and tune-ups. Check for brakes that are getting noisy or soft, as well as lights that have gone out or battery terminals that are corroded. Even if you don't do the repairs yourself, you will understand why replacing them may be necessary.

If you don't know how, learn to check your own tire pressure, change your oil, and refill essential fluids. You should be able to change a tire or a windshield wiper, and check the coolant. Know when to put on cold weather tires and winterize your engine, and if chains are called for in your area, understand how to put them on.

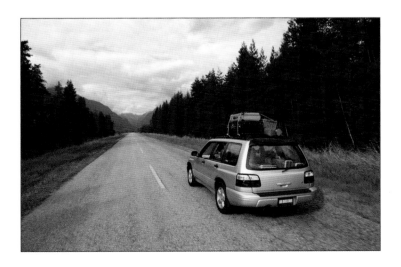

Never run your car on fumes. There should always be at least a half a tank of gas in your car. If you have an appropriate way to store it, consider keeping a two-week supply of fuel available for your car.

For some people, their car is an extension of their living room, strewn with spare clothing, food wrappers, and forgotten detritus. Keep your car decluttered and ready to go. Your car should always carry the following items:

- Blanket
- Rain ponchos
- Flashlight
- Sunscreen and insect repellant
- Water and a few energy bars
- Cash: dollar bills and quarters for tolls, and a spare $20 tucked into the glove box
- Jumper cables
- Cat litter or sand for better tire traction
- Shovel and ice scraper
- Basic car tools, including a jack, lug wrench, tow chain, and spare parts
- A couple of pints of oil, duct tape, and a gallon of engine coolant
- Light sticks and road flares
- An empty gas can

Your Go-Pack

Everyone in the family should have a go-pack ready in case of an emergency. If conditions call for concern, grab your pack and set it next to the door.

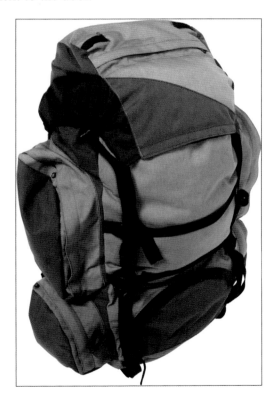

This kit should include:

- A three-day supply of food items containing protein, such as nuts and energy bars
- A three-day supply of water
- Basic toiletries, such as deodorant, toothpaste, etc.
- Spare eyeglasses
- Emergency blankets
- Warm clothes, gloves, a hat, closed-toe shoes, a jacket, and an extra change of clothes
- An LED headlamp
- Cell phone chargers (one for the car and one for wall outlets)
- Flashlights and extra batteries
- Battery powered AM/FM radio
- First aid kit and necessary medications
- Cash
- Some form of entertainment: books, cards, or games

Traveling Sensibly

If you know a hurricane is coming and you know where you plan to seek shelter, you may be able to leave before the roads are jammed with cars. I would much rather leave and find out that I can go home than sit in long lines of traffic with all the other procrastinators.

But some situations come on quickly. Uncertain weather conditions may cause you to hesitate. A last-minute decision to leave may put you on the road in a lot of traffic. Keep morale up and your patience in check. You may be in your car for quite a while, and may even end up sleeping overnight in it. Plan good music and other entertainment, and make sure you have snacks and plenty of water before you set out.

Plan your route, and check it with the latest traffic and weather advisories. The main roads may be jammed, so seek alternative roads before you need them to make sure they will provide a good escape route. Have paper maps in the car, along with your GPS, just in case you lose signal strength.

Make sure you tell someone what time you are leaving, what route you are taking, and the location of your final destination. Then stick to it. If you find you cannot get to your next location, check in and update someone. If you become stranded, stay with

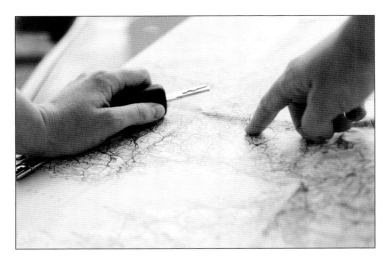

the car! It will provide adequate warmth and shelter until you can get assistance.

Signaling for Help

When it's time to get out, conditions may not be favorable. Plan ahead and know how to help others find you in case you get stranded.

- Notify friends or family of what time you are leaving, your planned route, and your expected destination. If you break down or are stuck, stay with the car.
- Make sure you have a phone charger for use in your car. Your phone can be used to track your location and help searchers find you.
- If you become stranded in the car, raise the trunk hood. This will indicate to passersby that you need assistance. Or carry a brightly colored flag to tie onto your antenna or luggage rack.
- If you are stranded in a remote area, set flares or build small fires to alert searchers of your presence.
- A flashlight or reflective material such as a mirror may help others locate you.
- Anything that makes a loud noise may also be useful. A whistle or an air horn requires much less energy and will travel much farther than your shouting.

Where to Go

While I admire the people who help to provide food and public shelter in an emergency, I can't help but think of shelters as for those who are totally unprepared. If you have thought things out, you already know where to go in an emergency and have made provisions to get there. Avoid public shelters, if at all possible.

Find a location that is within a distance that can be reached on one tank of gas. If everyone is on the roads, gas stations may have long lines or even run out of fuel. Make reciprocal arrangements with friends or family, or know the name of a hotel, a campground, or a bed and breakfast away from the

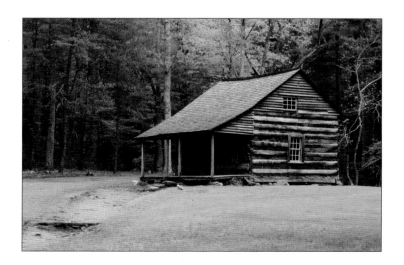

main highway that you can call as soon as you know you need it. If you are traveling with animals, make sure they accept pets. If you are traveling to a cabin or a second home, make sure that you have left it ready for last-minute visitors and stocked with extra sleeping bags, food, and water.

Useful Terms for Preppers

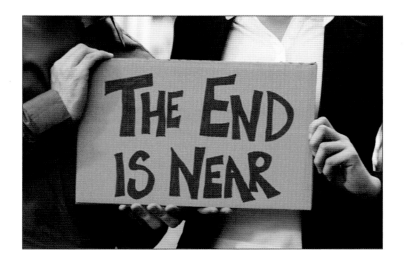

ABAO: All Bets Are Off

Bug-In Bag (BIB): A pack filled with everything you need for staying safe and staying put

Bug Out (BO): To hurriedly retreat to a safe location when threatened with imminent danger, (as in **Bug-Out Bag (BOB)**, **Bug-Out Location (BOL)**, **or Bug-Out Vehicle (BOV)**

Cache: Backup supplies hidden where you can readily obtain them during an emergency

Caldera: Enormous volcanic craters formed during an eruption. Explosive calderas can release enough debris to cause immense destruction and lower temperatures worldwide

Carrington Event: A powerful solar storm (same as CME and EMP)

CDC: Center for Disease Control

COMSEC: Communications Security

Coronal Mass Ejection (CME): Solar flares

DHS: Department of Homeland Security

DLP: Defense of Life and Property

Electromagnetic Pulse (EMP): A pulse that fries electronic devices

Everyday Carry (EDC): The bag you carry everywhere as a precaution

Extinction Level Event (ELE): An event that could cause human life to be exterminated

FEMA: Federal Emergency Management Agency

FUD: Fear, Uncertainty, and Doubt

Get–Home Bag (GHB): A kit to get you home during a disaster, should you happen to be away

Get Out Of Dodge (GOOD): To evacuate

Golden Horde: The mass of unprepared people fleeing or searching for shelter during a catastrophic event

ILT: Immediately Life Threatening

Isolated Retreat: A private shelter

MRE: Meal Ready to Eat

MSM: Mainstream Media

NVG: Night Vision Goggles

OPSEC: Operational Security

Pollyana: A person who refuses to believe evidence of TEOT-WAWKI

Prep: To prepare

Prepper: A person who prepares for disaster, and who seeks to maintain self-sufficiency during a catastrophe

Preps: Preparations

SERE: Survival, Evasion, Resistance, and Escape

Sheeple: Synonymous with Pollyana and Zombie

Shelter in Place (SIP): To shelter in your home, as opposed to bugging out

SHTF: Sh★t Hits The Fan

Survivalist: A highly skilled person able to survive in the worst situations

TEOTWAWKI: The End Of The World As We Know It

Without Rule of Law (WROL): Anarchy

WSHTF: When Sh★t Hits The Fan

You're On Your Own (YOYO): When government services and utilities cease to function and provide assistance

Zombie: Synonymous with Pollyana and Sheeple

Prepper Resources

There are many, many resources on the web for emergency products, food, and lighting. These are a few of my favorites:

Shelf Reliance
691 South Auto Mall Dr.
American Fork, UT 84003
801-756-9902
www.shelfreliance.com

The Wise Food Supply Company
8899 S. 700 E.
Sandy, UT 84070
888-406-2080
www.wisefoodsupply.com

Solar Oven Society
1754 Terrace Dr.
Roseville, MN 55113
612-623-4700
www.solarovens.org

Lodge Manufacturing
South Pittsburg, TN
423-837-7181
www.lodgemfg.com

Emergency Essentials
653 N. 1500 W.
Orem, UT 84057
800-999-1863
www.beprepared.com

SOS Survival Products
15705 Strathern St., #11
Van Nuys, CA 91406
800-479-7998
www.sosproduct.com

Grainger
800-323-0620
www.grainger.com

Brunton Outdoor
2255 Brunton Ct.
Riverton, WY 82501
307-857-4700
www.bruntonoutdoor.com

eGear
Revere Supply Company
7720 Philips Hwy.
Jacksonville, FL 32256
877-738-3738
www.egear.com

Yellowstone Trading Company
P.O. Box 3235
Bozeman, MT 59772
406-586-8248
www.yellowstonetrading.com

SproutPeople
170 Mendell St.
San Francisco, CA 94124
877-777-6887
www.sproutpeople.com

Notes